Handbook *of* Nutritional Support

Handbook *of* Nutritional Support

Alan Buchman, MD, MSPH, FACP, FACN
Associate Professor of Medicine
University of Texas Houston Health Science Center
Houston, Texas

Pediatric Section with
William J. Klish, MD
Professor of Pediatrics
Head, Pediatric Gastroenterology and Clinical Nutrition
Baylor College of Medicine
Houston, Texas

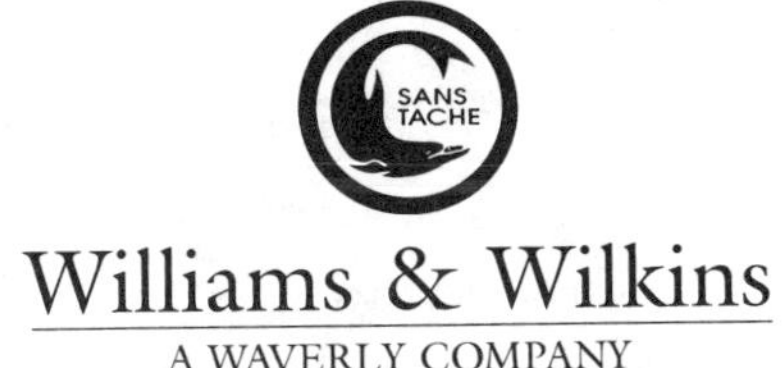

BALTIMORE • PHILADELPHIA • LONDON • PARIS • BANGKOK
BUENOS AIRES • HONG KONG • MUNICH • SYDNEY • TOKYO • WROCLAW

Editor: Jonathan W. Pine, Jr.
Managing Editor: Lynn Johnston
Marketing Manager: Daniell T. Griffin
Production Coordinator: Marette Magargle-Smith
Project Editor: Susan Rockwell
Typesetter: Peirce Graphic Services
Printer and Binder: Vicks Lithograph

351 West Camden Street
Baltimore, Maryland 21201-2436 USA

Rose Tree Corporate Center
1400 North Providence Road
Building II, Suite 5025
Media, Pennsylvania 19063-2043 USA

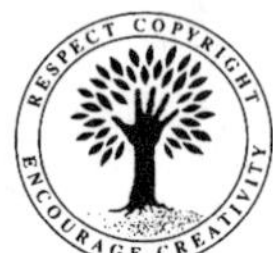

Accurate indications, adverse reactions and dosage schedules for drugs are provided in this book, but it is possible that they may change. The reader is urged to review the package information data of the manufacturers of the medications mentioned.

Printed in the United States of America

Library of Congress Cataloging-in-Publication Data

Buchman, Alan L.
Handbook of nutritional support / Alan L. Buchman.
p. cm.
Includes index.
ISBN 0-683-30238-8
1. Dietetics—Handbooks, manuals, etc. 2. Diet therapy—Handbooks, manuals, etc. 3. Nutrition—Handbooks, manuals, etc.
I. Title.
RM217.2.B78 1997
615.8′54—DC21 97–5928
CIP

The publishers have made every effort to trace the copyright holders for borrowed material. If they have inadvertently overlooked any, they will be pleased to make the necessary arrangements at the first opportunity.

To purchase additional copies of this book, call our customer service department at (800) 638-0672 or fax orders to (800) 447-8438. For other book services, including chapter reprints and large quantity sales, ask for the Special Sales department.

Canadian customers should call (800) 665-1148, or fax (800) 665-0103. For all other calls originating outside of the United States, please call (410) 528-4223 or fax us at (410) 528-8550.

Visit Williams & Wilkins on the Internet: http://www.wwilkins.com or contact our customer service department at custserv@wwilkins.com. Williams & Wilkins customer service representatives are available from 8:30 am to 6:00 pm, EST, Monday through Friday, for telephone access.

97 98 99 00
1 2 3 4 5 6 7 8 9 10

Preface

This handbook arose out of the need to educate the housestaff and attending physicians at the Baylor College of Medicine and The Methodist Hospital in the principles of nutritional assessment, recognition of the need for nutritional intervention, and the provision of nutritional support. Since its advent in the late 1960s, specialized nutritional support has become considerably more complex, as additional metabolic and technical information is accumulated. It has become exceedingly important that health care professionals, including physicians, pharmacists, nurses, dietitians, and trainees in each of these disciplines engaged in the delivery of nutritional support become properly educated in its use to ensure expected outcomes delivered in a cost effective manor with a limitation of complications.

The handbook is written in an outline format and follows a "cook book" approach to nutritional assessment, and provision of appropriate nutritional support with monitoring of goals and complications in adult and pediatric patients. Special sections for disease-specific nutrition and pregnancy are included. The handbook is intended as a guidebook for daily use, rather than as a reference textbook for the physiological basis of therapy. Where required, however, more extensive discussion is provided. References are provided for controversial issues, or issues for which additional information is beyond that necessary for routine patient care.

Alan Buchman, MD, MSPH

Acknowledgments

ADULT SECTION

The author acknowledges Stanley Dudrick, MD, Cindy Bloss, MS, RPH, BCNSP; Carolyn Moore, RD, PhD; Linda Pataki, RD, CNSD, CDE; Sonia Thomas, RN, BSN; Kirsh Jeejeebhoy, MD; Bill Byrne, MD; and Al Davies, MD, PhD, for their countless hours of manuscript review, comments, and suggestions. Patrick Reardon, MD, contributed to the section on central venous catheter insertion (with accompanying illustrations). The illustrations accompanying the indirect calorimetry were modified from those supplied by Sensormedics Inc., Yorba Linda, CA, with permission. The author is also indebted to Laurie Reyen, RN, Donald Yeough, RN, and William Guss, PharmD, for materials and reference materials supplied in helping to develop this book, nursing protocols, and TPN/enteral order forms for use at the Baylor College of Medicine and its affiliated institutions. I also thank Joan Ulrich, RD, for her helpful advice, and my mentor, Marvin Ament, MD, for much of what I have learned.

PEDIATRIC SECTION

The authors thank the Nutrition Support Team at Texas Children's Hospital and in particular Sarah Phillips, MS, RD; Theresa Reed, RN; and Robert Shulman, MD, for their help in preparing this section. The authors also thank Bill Byrne, MD, for his helpful review, comments, and suggestions.

Contents

CHAPTER 2
Nutritional Requirements 11

CHAPTER 3
Parenteral Nutrition 17

CHAPTER 7
Assessing the Efficacy of Nutritional Therapy 97

CHAPTER 8
Disease-Specific Nutrition 101

APPENDIX 1
Tables 000

CHAPTER 1

Nutritional Assessment

It is important to realize that no *single* test can be used as a completely reliable indicator of nutritional status. Proper nutritional assessment should evaluate anthropometric and laboratory data and should include an adequate history and physical examination. Every hospitalized patient should have basic nutritional assessment within 48 hours of admission and every 10 days thereafter.

HISTORY AND PHYSICAL EXAMINATION (SEE APPENDIX 1, TABLE 1)

History

- Unusual dietary habits
- Medications/vitamin and mineral supplementation
- Change in hair color or texture
- Poor night vision
- Dysgeusia
- Dysphagia/odynophagia
- Abdominal pain—distention
- Diarrhea
- Bone pain
- Muscle pain, cramps, or twitching
- Numbness, parathesias in extremities
- Fatigue
- Diminished mental activity
- Weakness or loss of strength

Physical Examination

- Hair loss, texture
- Keratomalacia
- Cheilosis
- Glossitis
- Red tongue
- Parotid enlargement
- Dentition

- Skin rash, petechiae bruising
- Muscle wasting
- Hepatomegaly
- Edema
- Peripheral neuropathy
- Assess gastrointestinal function
  May be affected by malnutrition alone or by primary gastrointestinal disease. Determine the functional status of the gastrointestinal tract, including gastric emptying and intestinal/colonic transit.

ANTHROPOMETRICS

Ideal Body Weight

Adult Females

100 lb (45 kg) for the first 60 inches (152 cm) + 5 lbs (2.3 kg) for every inch > 60.

Adult Males

106 lb (48 kg) for the first 60 inches (152 cm) + 6 lbs (2.7 kg) for every inch > 60.

Further information may be found in Appendix 1, Table 2.

Percent of Usual or Ideal Body Weight

Significant potential for malnutrition:

(a) >5% weight loss in 1 month
(b) >7.5% weight loss in 3 months
(c) >10% weight loss in 6 months

Preferred Body Weight (For Obese) Patients = (ABW − IBW) (0.25) + IBW

ABW = actual body weight
IBW = ideal body weight

	Usual or IBW (%)
Mild malnutrition	85–90
Moderate malnutrition	75–84
Severe malnutrition	< 74

The minimal survival weight is 48–55% of IBW (1).

Adjusted Body Weight for Amputation

Measured weight − % amputation

Corrections for Amputation	
Entire arm	6.5%
Upper arm	3.5%
Hand	0.8%

Forearm with hand	3.1%
Forearm without hand	2.5%
Entire leg	18.6%
Foot	1.8%

Mid-Arm Muscle Circumference (MAMC)

MAMC (cm) = MAC (cm) − 3.14 (triceps skin fold in cm)

- Assess skeletal mass
- Compare with normal values (Appendix 1, Table 3)
  - < 5th%—depletion
  - 5–25th%—at risk for depletion
  - < 85th%—at risk for obesity
- Not routinely used because of operator-dependent (variability), unreliable indicator of short-term response to nutritional therapy. Primarily for use in population studies.

Muscle Function

Muscle function testing is not usually useful as an initial screening tool but may be useful in serial assessments. Improvements in hand grip strength measured by dynamometry or respiratory muscle strength (peak inspiratory and expiratory pressures) are useful (see Appendix 1, Tables 4 and 5).

Triceps Skin Fold Thickness

- Assess fat stores
- Compare with normal values (Appendix 1, Tables 6 and 7)
- Not routinely used because of operator-dependent (variability), unreliable indicator of short-term response to nutritional therapy. Primarily for use in population studies.

Methods of Measuring Skinfolds and Circumferences (See Fig. 3.3)

Skinfolds

1. Arrive at the anatomic site as defined (the midpoint between the acromial and olecranon processes of the scapula and the ulna, respectively. The arm should hang relaxed at the patient's side).
2. Lift the skin and fat layer from the underlying tissue by grasping the tissue with the thumb and forefinger.
3. Apply calipers about 1 cm distal from the thumb and forefinger, midway between the apex and the base of the skinfold.
4. Continue to support the skinfold with the thumb and forefinger for the duration of the measurement.
5. After 2 to 3 seconds of caliper application, read skinfold to the nearest 0.5 mm.
6. Measurements are then made in triplicate until readings within ± 1.0 mm; results are then averaged.

Circumferences

1. The tape should be maintained in a horizontal position touching the skin and following the contours of the limb, but not compressing the underlying tissue.
2. Measurements should be made to the nearest millimeter, in triplicate, as previously described for skinfolds.

LABORATORY MEASUREMENTS

Nitrogen Balance

➢ Often helpful in determining whether sufficient protein and/or calories are being provided.

$$N_I(g) = \frac{\text{g protein/d}}{6.25}$$

The average protein is approximately 15% nitrogen, hence 6.25 is used as the denominator.

To calculate nitrogen output:

➢ Use 24-hour total urine nitrogen (TUN) or urine urea nitrogen (UUN). TUN is preferable.

UUN represents, on the average, only 80–90% of TUN, although the range can be as great as 12–112%. This may result in variations of up to 12 g (2).

Increased nonurea nitrogen (including uric acid, ammonia, creatinine and other minor compounds) loss may occur during "stress," especially in major burns (3) or a change in hydration status.

Avoid pH adjustments and heating of urine samples because this may lead to falsely low TUN (4).

➢ Daily fecal N losses in patients without malabsorption or protein-losing enteropathy during parenteral nutrition ranges between 0.3–0.8 g/day or approximately 8 mg/kg/day.

➢ Integumental losses, in the absence of large wounds or burns, range between 7 mg/kg/day for women and 8 mg/kg/day for men (5)

$$\text{Nitrogen balance} = N_{\text{intake(I)}} - N_{\text{output (O)}}$$

or

$$N_I - (\text{UUN} + 4)$$

➢ For anabolism, + N balance of at least 4–6 g is required.

➢ Achievement of positive N balance requires not only sufficient protein or amino acids, but adequate calories as well.

➢ N retention does not necessarily indicate effective N utilization.

➢ Correct N balance for the change in nonprotein N in patients who have a change in blood urea nitrogen (BUN) during the urine collection:

$$\Delta \text{ Nonprotein nitrogen (g/d)} = [BUN_f - BUN_i) \times 0.6 \times BW_i + (BW_f - BW_i) \times BUN_f]/Day_f - Day_i)$$

i = initial BW = body weight (kg)
f = final BUN = g/L

Indirect Calorimetry

- Measures the basal energy expenditure (BEE) required to fuel basic life functions at rest in a neutral thermic environment, 10 or more hours after eating.
- Helpful in estimating caloric requirements, especially in patients who are significantly underweight or overweight, (with significant fluid retention) or significantly catabolic.
- BEE is estimated from known values of heat produced by the combustion of carbohydrate, fat, and protein and measurement of inspired O_2 and expired CO_2 using the Weir equation (6).

$$\text{kcal/d} = (3.941 \times VO_2\ [\text{L/day})] + (1.106 \times VCO_2\ [\text{L/day}]\ ) - (2.17 \times TUN[\text{g/day}]$$

VO_2 = O_2 consumption
VCO_2 = CO_2 production
TUN = total urine nitrogen (24 hr)

- Most typically, utilized in an open-circuit system in which patient breathes either ambient or oxygen-enriched air (via a ventilator or non-air leak face mask)

Mechanism

- In the nonventilated patient, a clear plastic hood, through which a stream of room air flows, is placed over the patient's head (Fig. 1.1). Alternatively, a mouth piece (into which patient inspires and expires) with a noseclip to avoid nasal inspiration/expiration can be used. For the ventilated patient, a vacuum line is interposed between the endotracheal tube and ventilator tube (Fig. 1.2). The expired gas is diluted and removed through the expiratory port of the hood or mouthpiece. The diluted air is passed through a volume-measuring device (for measurement of minute ventilation), through a mixing chamber (to achieve a steady concentration of inspired gases), and then through O_2 and CO_2 analyzers. In the ventilated patient, inspired and expired gases are sampled continuously at a constant rate.
- O_2 consumption and CO_2 production are calculated from measurements of inspired and expired gas and from minute ventilation. The difference in gas concentration between room air and exhaled air is multiplied by the gas flow rate through the system. The process is similar in a ventilated patient, except that a vacuum line is interposed. O_2 and CO_2 measurements are weighted according to the corresponding flow rate measured simultaneously by the pneumotach. A phase delay ensures that gas and flow measurements are appropriately matched.

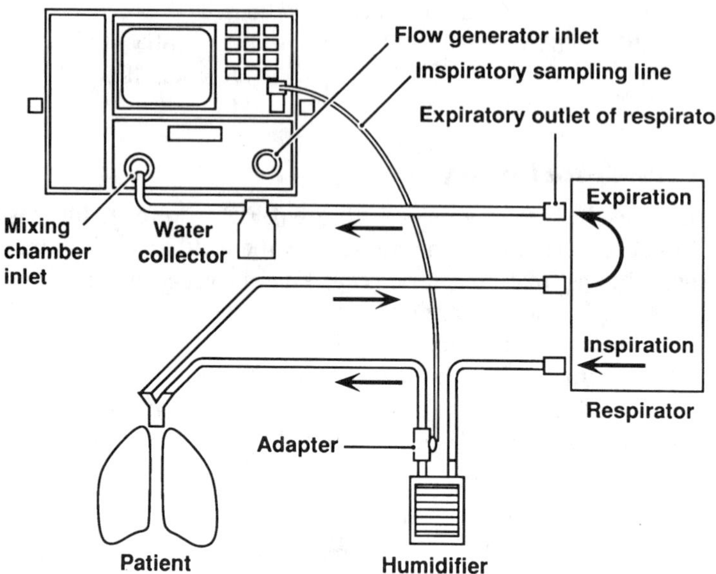

Figure 1.1.
Indirect calorimetry respiratory measurements for ventilated patient.

Procedure

- Usually requires about 30 minutes to perform, including a 10-minute equilibration period, in which the patient is allowed to become accustomed to the hood or mouthpiece/noseclip system to exclude a hyperventilation artifact and to allow for achievement of a steady state.
- Patient should be resting, but not asleep during the test period.
- There should be no interruption, such as medication dosing, eating, phlebotomy, or ventilator adjustments during the test period.
- Valid gas measurement cannot be obtained for patients who are receiving supplemental oxygen via non-airtight facemask, nasal cannula, or $> 60\%$ FiO_2. Even small fluctuations in inspired O_2 tension, commonly encountered in many mechanical ventilator systems, can markedly alter O_2 consumption measurement, especially when a high FiO_2 is used.
- VO_2 is usually 3–4 ml/min/kg in normal subjects, so any outlying values should be evaluated. For example, a patient in extreme pain or with head trauma who is hyperventilating, may have a VO_2 of 5–7 ml/min/kg. Incorrect values may be caused by leaks, inaccurate volume measurements, or unstable gas analyzers.

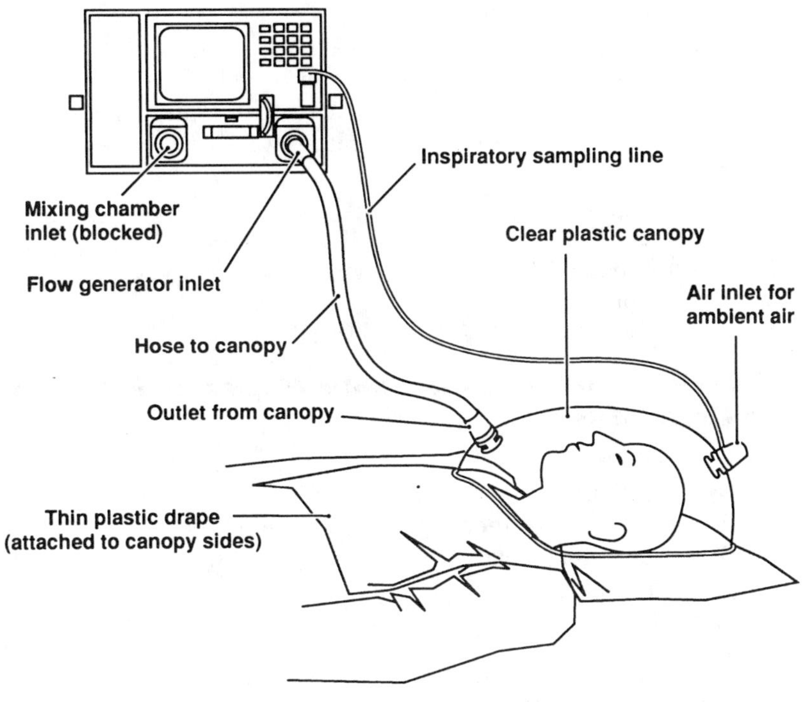

Figure 1.2.
Indirect calorimetry canopy measurements with room air.

- Consult individual factory technical manuals for information and other technical problems or calibration of the metabolic cart.
- Perform after a minimum of 6 hours fasting (preferably 8–12 hours). It is unnecessary to discontinue continuous feeding (enteral or parenteral) but keep in mind, the REE will then include the thermogenic effect of food. The thermogenic effect of food is on the order of 10% (7), although a range of 5–30% has been reported.
- Hypo- or hypermetabolism occur when measured REE varies more than 10% from that predicted using the Harris Benedict equations.
- Total energy expenditure includes an activity factor and the thermogenic response to food (either parenteral or enteral) and is thought to add approximately 20% to the REE for patients undergoing “usual” hospital treatment. Additional activity such as intense rehabilitation will increase caloric demands while a comatose patient will expend little energy for activity. The only rule is to use common sense, follow response to nutritional therapy, and repeat the indirect calorimetry at regular intervals if necessary.

Factors Affecting REE	
Height and weight	Pain
Age	Fever/hypothermia
Sex	Thermogenic effect of food
Medications	Sleep/awake

↑REE	↓REE
Caffeine	Beta blockers
Aspirin	Alpha blockers
Epinephrine	Narcotics
	Anesthesia

Situations In Which Metabolic Measurements May Be Unreliable

- $FiO_2 > 60\%$
- Hyperventilation
- Poor patient cooperation (agitated or sleeping)
- Bronchopleural fistula
- Trachea cuff leak
- PEEP, PEFR
- Tremor, seizures

Respiratory Quotient (RQ)

- Calculated by determining the ratio of expired CO_2 to inspired O_2

RQ > 1.0	Usually reflects nonsteady state, hyperventilation, or overfeeding
RQ = 1.0	Carbohydrate oxidation
RQ = 0.85	Mixed substrate "oxidation"
RQ = 0.70	Fat oxidation
RQ = 1.0 − 1.2	Lipogenesis
RQ = 0.67	Alcohol and ketone metabolism

- It is important to note whether the RQ is within physiologic range (0.7–1.3) and consistent with the patient's nutritional intake. For example, the RQ should be 0.7–0.8 (consistent with fat oxidation) in a patient whose sole nutritional intake has been D_5W for a week. Therefore, an RQ of ≥ 1.0 should be viewed with suspicion in such a patient.
- Errors may have been caused by technical problems, hyperventilation because the patient received an injection during the gas measurement, for instance, or the unrecorded administration or a large dextrose load.
- RQ may vary during hemo- or peritoneal dialysis (8)

Factors Increasing RQ
Hyperventilation
Metabolic acidosis
Overfeeding/lipogenesis

Exercise
Calibration errors or leaks in the metabolic cart

Visceral Proteins

Albumin

Normal (3.5–5.0 g/dL)
Mildly depleted (3.0–3.5 g/dL)
Moderately depleted (2.5–3.0 g/dL)
Severely depleted (< 2.5 g/dL)

- Poor indicator of short-term changes in visceral protein status and may be unreliable in some medical conditions.
- Non-nutritional factors may *elevate* albumin concentration: albumin infusion, dehydration, renal failure, anabolic steroids
- Non-nutritional factors may *depress* albumin concentration: pregnancy, severe burns, protein-losing enteropathy, nephrotic syndrome, edema, hepatic insufficiency, neoplastic disease, severe infections, trauma, or post surgery

Pre-Albumin

Normal (18–24 mg/dL)
Mildly depleted (16–18 mg/dL)
Moderately depleted (14–16 mg/dL)
Severely depleted (< 14 mg/dL)

- 1.9 day half life (9)
- More sensitive marker than albumin for assessing rapid nutritional changes, although subject to similar non-nutritional factors.
- May be elevated in renal failure and suppressed in hepatic failure.
- Pre-albumin and nitrogen balance measurement are the preferred parameters in the assessment of total body protein status.

Transferrin

Normal (200–250 mg/dL)
Mildly depleted (170–200 mg/dL)
Moderately depleted (140–170 mg/dL)
Severely depleted (< 140 mg/dL)

- May be elevated due to iron deficiency anemia, as an acute phase reactant, during pregnancy, or during the use of oral contraceptives.
- May be suppressed in renal and hepatic failure despite adequate protein status.
- Although a significant relationship exists between serum transferrin concentration and nutritional status, the variation in concentration may lend a greater usefulness in population studies rather than in the individual patient (11)

Retinol-Binding Protein

- Half life is 12 hours. Too short for practical value and no advantages over pre-albumin

Insulin-like Growth Factor-1

- Investigational (12)

Immune Function

Total Lymphocyte Count

Normal (1600–4000 per mm^3)
Mild depletion (1200–1600 per m^3)
Moderate depletion (800–1200 per m^3)
Severe depletion (< 800 per m^3)

- May be depressed by non-nutritional factors including chemotherapy, radiation therapy, glucocorticoids, and viral infections.

Delayed Hypersensitivity Skin Tests

- Commonly used antigens include mumps, trichophyton, candida, tetanus and intermediate strength purified protein derivative (PPD). A 5-mm response or greater at 24–48 hours is considered a positive response.
- May be affected by non-nutritional factors including corticosteroids, T-cell deficiency, cancer, immunosuppressive medications.

REFERENCES

1. University of Minnesota Laboratory of Physiological Hygiene. The Biology of Starvation, 1950.
2. Konstantinides FN, Konstantinides NN, Li JC, et al. Urinary urea nitrogen: too insensitive for calculating nitrogen balance studies in surgical clinical nutrition. JPEN 1991;15:189–193.
3. Bell SJ, Molner JA, Kraske WS. Prediction of total urinary nitrogen from urea nitrogen of burned patients. J Am Diet Assoc 1985;85:1100–1104.
4. Konstantinides FN, Maga VK, Herman BA, et al. Routine laboratory preparation of twenty-four-hour urine samples for nitrogen determinations induces false low total urinary nitrogen (TUN) levels. JPEN 1992;16:33S.
5. Calloway DH, Odell AC, Margen S. Sweat and miscellaneous nitrogen losses in human balance studies. J Nutr 1971;101:775–786.
6. Weir JB. New methods for calculating metabolic rate with special reference to protein metabolism. J Physiol 1949;109:1–9.
7. Elwyn DH, Kinney JM, Askanazi J. Energy expenditure in surgical patients. Surg Clin North Am 1981;61:545–549.
8. Sigler MH, Skutches CL, Teehan BP, et al. Acetate and energy metabolism during hemodialysis. Kidney Intl Sup 1983;24:597–610.
9. Socolow EL, Woeber KA, Purdy RH, et al. Preparation of I131—labeled human serum prealbumin and its metabolism in normal and sick patients. J Clin Invest 1965; 44:1600–1609.
10. Ingenbleek Y, van den Schrieck HG, de Nayer P, et al. Albumin, transferrin and the thyroxine-binding prealbumin/retinal-binding protein (TBPA-RBP) complex in assessment of malnutrition. Clin Chem Acta 1975;63:61–67.
11. Ryan JA Jr, Page CP. Intra jejunal feeding: development and current status. JPEN 1984;8:523–528.
12. Am J Clin Nutr 1989;50:962–969.

CHAPTER 2

Nutritional Requirements

FLUID REQUIREMENTS

Maintenance

1500 ml + 20 ml/kg for every kg > 20 kg

- Increases by 10% for every 1°C of fever.
- May be decreased significantly in cirrhosis, congestive heart failure, pulmonary edema, ARDS, or renal failure.

Replacement Fluid

- Extraneous fluid losses (e.g., nasogastric or enteric suction, biliary or fistula drainage, diarrhea or emesis) should be replaced with a *separate* intravenous solution in amounts equal to measured losses every 8 hours. Fluid retention may also occur during TPN. Weight gain of > 1–2 kg/wk is probably related to fluid retention.
- Avoid the use of TPN to replace extraneous fluid and electrolyte losses because of the significant extra expense. Replace with common intravenous electrolyte solutions when possible.
- See Appendix 1, Table 14 for body fluid electrolyte concentrations

CALORIC REQUIREMENTS

Actual calorie requirements can only be estimated in the absence of direct calorimetry. The formulas shown and indirect calorimetry are helpful in making the appropriate estimations.

Harris Benedict Equation

- Estimates basal metabolic rate (BMR).

Males: 66.47 + 13.75 (wt,kg) + 5 (ht,cm) − 6.76 (age,yr)
Females: 655.1 + 9.56 (wt,kg) + 1.85 (ht,cm) − 4.68 (age,yr)

- Multiply result by 1.2–1.5 "activity" factors to account for physical activity and disease stress.

- Derived from studies on young *healthy* adults, so it is often inaccurate in the hospital setting, especially in critically ill patients. For instance, when the REE is measured in trauma, or with infected or mechanically ventilated patients using indirect calorimetry, values of 70–140% of those predicted using the Harris Benedict equation have been described (1, 2). Studies in acutely ill surgical patients show that the Harris Benedict equation may overestimate caloric requirements by an average of 59% (3). Each degree (°C) increase in body temperature increases the REE by 7–13% (4–6). Mechanical ventilation and medications such as barbiturates, muscle relaxants such as curare and pancuronium and beta blockers such as propranolol may decrease metabolic rate. Metabolic rate is usually increased significantly in patients with major burns because significant energy must be used to maintain body temperature. However, the REE usually declines during convalescence. Care must be taken not to undernourish or overfeed patients.

Indirect Calorimetry

- Measures resting energy expenditure (REE).
- Add ~ 20% for activity.

Caloric Requirements by Weight (IBW) or Preferred Body Weight

Maintenance (30–35 kcal/kg)

- Non-hospitalized patients usually require 25–30 kcal/kg.

Rebuild Lean Body Mass (35–40 kcal/kg)

- In patients who are severely underweight, REE is often depressed and actual body weight should be used in preference to IBW in the initial days of nutritional support to avoid refeeding syndrome (hypophosphatemia).

Calorie:Nitrogen Ratio

- Sufficient non-protein calories (i.e., dextrose, lipid) must be administered to enable the efficient use of protein synthesis and to prevent the catabolism of skeletal muscle and exogenous amino acids for use as a calorie support with subsequent development of kwashiorkor. Protein provides 5.65 kcal/g. However, when the water dilution of protein and the energy lost in the form of urea are considered, protein supplies only **1 kcal/g**. Therefore, protein becomes a poor and expensive glucose source when sufficient dextrose calories are not provided.
- The optimal non-protein calorie:nitrogen ratio is 150–200:1.
- See Appendix 1, Table 9 for ratios in standard TPN solutions.

PROTEIN REQUIREMENTS

Protein requirements can only be estimated in the absence of nitrogen balance determination.

- 0.6–0.8 g/kg/day in healthy human.
- 0.8–1.0 g/kg/day in hospitalized patient.
- 1.1–1.5 g/kg/day for protein repletion.
- $>$ 1.5 g/kg/day only in severe burns and protein losing enteropathy. Excess protein will not result in greater tissue synthesis.
- 0.55 g/kg/day minimum in renal failure or hepatic failure in the absence of dialysis (7).
- Add 6–9 g/day for hemodialysis, including CHD and CVVHD (1.0–1.2 g/kg/d) (8, 9).
- Add 12–16 g/day for peritoneal dialysis (1.2–1.4 g/kg/d) (10–12).

Specialized Amino Acid Products

See Appendix 1, Table 23 for product composition.

Branched Chain Amino Acids

High Branched Chain (HBC) Formula

This formula is possibly of benefit in severely catabolic patients with multiple trauma, sepsis or multiorgan failure syndrome and lactic acidosis and hyperglycemia. Clinical efficacy has *not* been demonstrated. Therefore, this formulation should not be used outside of a research protocol.

Elevated Branched Chain (BCAA)/Low Aromatic Amino Acid (AAA) Formula

The use of this formula is predicated by the false neurotransmitter theory of James et al. (13) and the observation that serum ammonia concentration is often elevated in hepatic encephalopathy. The false neurotransmitter theory assumes that the imbalance between plasma BCAA (leucine, isoleucine and valine) and AAA (tyrosine, phenylalanine and tryptophan) leads to an increased influx of the AAA into the brain. BCAA and AAA compete for the same amino acid transporter across the blood-brain barrier (BBB). Relative plasma concentration gradients determine those amino acids preferentially transported across the BBB. The relative increase in plasma AAA leads to increased AAA across the BBB and into the brain. The excessive amounts of these AAA are the precursors of "false neurotransmitters" such as octopamine and B-phenylethanolamine, which are thought to precipitate hepatic coma.

The therapeutic approach of using a high BCAA/low AAA-containing formula is an attempt to normalize the relative plasma amino acid concentrations. In addition, high BCAA/low AAA formulas provide substrates that bind ammonia:

$$\begin{array}{l}\text{valine} \rightarrow \text{succinate} \rightarrow \text{a-ketoglutarate}\\ \text{glutamine} \leftarrow \text{glutamate}\\ \quad\downarrow\\ \quad NH_3\end{array}$$

Leucine, in particular, stimulates protein synthesis and thereby possibly inhibits protein and peripheral muscle catabolism, thus generating less ammonia.

Although theoretically attractive, the clinical efficacy of high BCAA/low AAA formulas have not been conclusively demonstrated. Therefore, and because of the extra expense of this formulation, clear outcome goals in a specified time trial are necessary for its use; if efficacy is demonstrated in a given patient, the formula may be continued until it has been determined that the patient had improved to the point where use of standard amino acid formulas might be tolerated.

Renal Formula

This formulation consists of only essential amino acids. Histidine is considered an essential amino acid in renal failure. While theoretically beneficial, clinical studies have demonstrated no improvement in morbidity or mortality and no consistent decrease in urea generation when compared with standard amino acid solutions in equivalent amounts. At best, only small metabolic improvements may be noted. This formula therefore should not be used outside of a research protocol (14, 15). There may be benefit from using specialized renal formulas during CAVH when nitrogenous wastes are not removed. However, these formulas have not been studied in randomized-controlled trials during CAVH.

FAT REQUIREMENTS

The minimum fat content of the diet is 2–4% of total calories consisting of linoleic acid. That is to prevent *essential fatty acid deficiency (EFAD).* Decreased serum linoleic acid concentration, an increase in ratio of 5,8,11 eicosatrienoic acid to arachodonic acid to > 0.4. Increased palmitoleic and oleic acid concentrations may also be found. Scaly skin rash, hair loss, hepatomegaly and possibly anemia, thrombocytopenia, osteoporosis, and decreased wound healing may occur. Most lipid emulsions are typically 50% linoleic acid. Medium chain triglycerides (MCT) do not provide essential fats. Linolenic acid has not been conclusively demonstrated to be essential in humans because only a single case report of a child developing a neuropathy associated with linolenic acid deficiency has been reported. Biochemical evidence of EFAD may occur within 2 weeks of the provision of lipid-free TPN although clinical deficiency does not develop for about 6 weeks.

ELECTROLYTE, VITAMIN, AND TRACE ELEMENT REQUIREMENTS

Requirements may vary depending on underlying pathology and the need to replace deficient states or to prevent toxicity. For most patients receiving parenteral nutrition, standard electrolyte, vitamin and trace element solutions will provide daily patient needs if adequate calories are infused (see Appendix 1, Tables 4, 6, 10, 26, and 27). Likewise, most enteral products are designed to meet the RDA for electrolytes, vitamins, and trace elements if adequate amounts to provide optimal caloric intake are provided. It is important to include electrolyte content such as sodium and potassium bound to medication in the calculation of daily intake (see Appendix 1, Tables 31–34).

Electrolyte Abnormalities

- May result from inadequate replacement of body losses (see Appendix 1, Table 14).
- As protein synthesis occurs with refeeding, potassium and phosphorus requirements will increase.
- Extreme hyperglycemia will cause a pseudohyponatremia.
- Increased endogenous or exogenous insulin will cause a decrease in serum potassium and possibly magnesium.
- See Appendix 1, Table 15 for signs and symptoms of electrolyte abnormalities.

Trace Element Abnormalities

- May result from inadequate replacement of body losses (e.g., zinc and selenium lost in diarrhea) or excessive replacement (e.g., copper during severe cholestasis).
- See Appendix 1, Table 16 for signs and symptoms of trace element abnormalities.

Vitamin Abnormalities

- Unusual.
- May result from excessive replacement during states of inadequate metabolism/excretion (e.g., vitamin A in renal failure).
- See Appendix 1, Table 17 for signs and symptoms of vitamin deficiency/toxicity.
- Required *water soluble* vitamins in humans include thiamine (B_1), riboflavin (B_2), niacin (B_3), pantothenic acid (B_5), pyridoxin (B_6), cyanocobalamin (B_{12}), folic acid, ascorbic acid (C), and biotin.
- Required *fat soluble* vitamins include retinol (A), calciferol (D), tocopherol (E), and phytonadione (K).

References

1. Carlson M, Nordenstrom J, Hedenstierne. Clinical implications of continuous measurement of energy expenditure in mechanically ventilated patients. Clin Nutr 1984;3:103–110.
2. Weissman C, Kemper M, Askenazi J, et al. Resting metabolic rate of the critically ill patient: measured versus predicted. Anesthesiology 1986;64:673–679.
3. Mann S, Westenskow DR, Houtchens BA. Measured and predicted caloric expenditure in the acutely ill. Crit Care Med 1985;13:173–177.
4. Paige DM. Clinical Nutrition. 2nd ed. St. Louis: Mosby, 1988:363.
5. Shils ME, Olson JA, Shike M. Modern Nutrition. 8th ed. Philadelphia: Lee and Febiger, 1988:826.

6. Kiney JM, Furst P, Elwyn OH, et al. The Intensive Care Patients. In: Kinney JM, Jeejeebhoy K, Hill GL, Owen OE, eds. Nutrition and Metabolism in Patient Care. Philadelphia: WB Saunders, 1988:658.
7. Eastwood M. Dietary fiber and the risks of cancer. Nutr Rev 1987;39:193.
8. Kopple JD, Swendseid ME, Shinaberger JH, et al. The free end band amino acids removed by hemodialysis. Trans Am Soc Artif Int Organ 1973:4:309.
9. Davies Sp. Amino acid clearance and daily losses in patients with acute renal failure treated by continuous arteriovenous hemodialysis. Crit Care Med 1991;19:1510.
10. Berlyne GM, Lee HA, Giordano C, et al. Amino acid loss in peritoneal dialysis. Lancet 1967:1339–1341.
11. Kopple JD, Monteon FJ, Shaib JK. Effect of energy intake on nitrogen metabolism in nondialyzed patients with chronic renal failure. Kidney Int 1986;29:734.
12. Blumenkrantz MJ, Kopple JD, Moran JK, et al. Metabolic balance studies and dietary protein requirements in patients undergoing continuous ambulatory peritoneal dialysis. Kidney Int 1982;21:849.
13. James JH, Ziparo V, Jeppsson B, et al. Hyperammonaemia, plasma aminoacid imbalance, and blood-brain aminoacid transport: a unified theory of portal-systemic encephalopathy. Lancet 1979;2:772.
14. Feinstein EI, Blumenkrantz. Clinical and metabolic responses to parenteral nutrition in acute renal failure: A controlled double-blind study. Medicine 1981;60:124.
15. Druml W. Nutritional support in acute renal failure. Clin Nutr 1993;12:196.

CHAPTER 3

Parenteral Nutrition

INDICATIONS

In general, total parenteral nutrition is indicated if the small intestine is dysfunctional, obstructed, or inaccessible or the colon is severely dysfunctional or obstructed, and this condition is expected to continue a minimum of 7 days.

Specific Indications

a. *Intractable vomiting*—e.g., severe acute pancreatitis, hyperemesis gravidarum, chemotherapy.
b. *Severe diarrhea*— (>500 ml stool) or malabsorption, e.g., severe, acute flare of inflammatory bowel disease, graft versus host disease, severe sprue or sprue-like conditions, short bowel syndrome (< 50–60 cm of remaining bowel), radiation enteritis with weight loss.
c. *Severe mucositis/esophagitis*—e.g., chemotherapy, graft versus host disease.
d. *Ileus*—e.g., severe trauma/major abdominal surgery or pseudo-obstruction, when enteral nutrition, including feeding jejunostomy cannot be used for at least 7 days.
e. *Small bowel or colon obstruction*—e.g., cancer, adhesions, infectious, pseudo-obstruction.
f. *"Bowel Rest"*—e.g., enterocutaneous or entero-enteric fistula, anastomotic leak, Crohn's disease of small intestine.
g. *Preop*—e.g., only in cases of *severe* malnutrition, otherwise surgery should not be delayed.
   - *Intraoperative* parenteral nutrition is relatively contraindicated; there is no demonstrated efficacy and should intraoperative fluid resuscitation be required the risk of inadvertently increasing the parenteral nutrition infusion rate could have potentially serious ramifications. Severe metabolic and/or electrolyte disturbances may occur rapidly in the perioperative period.
h. Parenteral nutrition is *not* indicated in patients who have a gastrointestinal tract capable of adequate nutrient absorption, whenever parenteral duration is expected to be less than 7 days, in mildly malnourished preop patients, in patients in whom parenteral nutrition is not desired by the patient or legal guardian, or in whom the disease prognosis is not improved by the use of parenteral nutrition. On the other

hand, the nutritional assessment for nutritional support should be considered within the first 24 hours; do not wait 7 days.

Central Parenteral Nutrition (CPN)

- The high osmolality (>900 mOsm) of most PN solutions requires administration into large veins with high blood flow in order to avoid phlebitis. The catheter tip should rest in the superior or inferior vena cava.
- To limit the risk of infection, a central venous catheter inserted solely for the use of PN should be used.

Peripheral Parenteral Nutrition (PPN)

- Should be provided to patients who require only short-term therapy (< 7–10 days) and can meet much but not all of their nutritional requirements via enteral means. This therapy may provide for some protein sparing.
- Because the solutions are hypertonic, thrombophlebitis of the site of administration is inevitable. Never use dextrose solutions of greater than 10% concentration or 900 mOsm.
- Hydrocortisone 10 mg and heparin 1000 units/l may prevent thrombophlebitis (1, 2). There are rare reports of heparin-induced thrombocytopenia.
- Hospital policy often precludes administration of intravenous medications into the same peripheral vein as parenteral nutrition known to cause phlebitis (acyclovir, aminoglycosides, amphotericin, erythromycin, high dose penicillins, phenytoin, potassium, vancomycin).

Intradialytic Parenteral Nutrition

- Intradialytic parenteral nutrition (IDPN) is indicated *only* in patients who are receiving chronic hemodialysis, have poor oral intake, and cannot be enterally fed or provided with central PN. Medicare regulations enacted in June 1987 are stringent on the proper indications. The medical record must demonstrate the patient has poor dietary intake, has lost > 10% of dry weight, has fat and peripheral muscle wasting, depressed serum albumin in addition to one or more of the diagnoses listed under indications for PN.
- IDPN is safe (3) if a moderate infusion rate is maintained and proper monitoring is performed. Typical infusion is a single liter and includes approximately 7 kcal/kg from dextrose, 1.6 g/kg of lipid emulsion, and 0.22 g/kg amino acids. The rate should be initiated at no more than 150 ml/hr to avoid profound hyperglycemia. The rate is then gradually increased so that the full liter can be infused during a 4-hour dialysis. The increased lipid as a percentage of total calories may be helpful in avoiding the hyperglycemia, although large triglyceride loads may not be handled well either. The superiority of an essential amino acid-containing formula over a mixed essential/nonessential amino acid-containing formula has not been demonstrated (4). Blood glucose monitoring should

be frequent during the infusion and at 30 and 60 minutes after the infusion to detect reactive hypoglycemia which may be more life-threatening than the hyperglycemia. If possible, some sweetened orange juice or other simple carbohydrate beverage should be provided 20–30 minutes after the infusion.

CONTRAINDICATIONS

PN may not be appropriate in hemodynamically unstable patients including those with hypovolemia, cardiogenic or septic shock; patients with severe pulmonary edema or fluid overload; anuria without dialysis or profound metabolic or electrolyte disturbances. Concentrated PN may be required for patients with overhydration.

COMPONENTS OF PARENTERAL NUTRITION

Central Venous Catheter

(See Appendix 1, Table 18)

- ➢ Catheter tip should rest in the superior or inferior vena cava and be documented by radiography before initiation of infusion.
- ➢ Double and triple lumen short-term catheters may be used if a dedicated PN line is unavailable. However, multi-lumen catheters carry a higher rate of sepsis than single lumen catheters. If multilumen catheters must be used, a designated PN port should be used. A pulmonary artery catheter (Swan-Ganz) is a violated line and should not be used for PN. Intrusion of a central venous catheter should be permitted only under emergency conditions (e.g., CPR). A catheter lumen reserved for PN should not be used for CVP monitoring, blood infusion, or drug therapy.
- ➢ The use of routine line changes/replacement is controversial. It remains unclear as to whether routine line change or replacement is associated with decreased infection risk. There are mechanical risks associated with replacement (5, 6).

Catheter Types

Short-term Catheters	Long-term Catheters
Triple, double, single lumen (ex. Arrow Cath, Cook Cath)	Tunneled silastic single and double lumen (Hickman, Broviac)
Cordis	Percutaneous inserted central catheter (PICC lines)
Swan Ganz (pulmonary artery catheters)	Subcutaneous infusion ports
Arterial lines	

Catheter Insertion

Site Choice

The subclavian vein is the preferred route for central venous access for TPN (Fig. 3.1). This site allows for access to the central circulation and provides an immobile area for catheter fixation. This not only makes it more comfortable for the patient, but the broad, flat surface allows for placement of a truly occlusive dressing. This may be difficult to achieve in some patients.

The internal jugular vein is the next most frequently accessed site. The neck is much more mobile, however, and lines placed at these sites are more uncomfortable for the patient. The rounded surface of the neck with its muscular contours makes achieving a truly occlusive dressing more difficult as well.

The femoral vein site may be associated with an increased incidence of infection. The skin puncture site is frequently at the groin crease, where the skin flora has a greater concentration of potentially pathogenic organisms. This is a warm, moist area with a great deal of movement. This makes maintenance of an occlusive dressing very difficult. Infusion of concentrated solutions into these veins may lead to iliofemoral vein thrombosis with its subsequent risk of pulmonary embolism. This site should almost never be accessed for TPN if other more preferable sites are available.

Technique

Triple-Lumen Catheter

- Informed consent.
- The operator should don cap, mask, sterile gown, and sterile gloves.

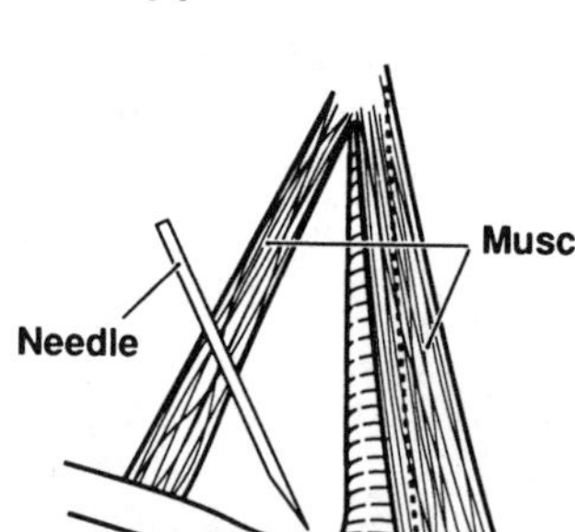

Figure 3.1.
Supraclavicular approach.

- Place patient in supine position in Trendelenburg position with head turned away from the catherization site.
- Prep skin with povidone-iodine or 2% chlorhexidine from the sternum to the lateral edge of the chest and from the jaw line to 8–10 cm below the clavicle.
- Use patient's nondominant side if possible.
- Use sterile towel or drapes to provide a sterile field.
- Determine the length of the catheter to be inserted so that the tip resides within the SVC if possible (never in the heart). The external marker for the junction of the SVC and the right atrium is at the "Angle of Louis" where the manubrium and sternal body meet. Then place the catheter along the track of the vein until the guidewire is met. The distance along the catheter may be measured at this point with the markers on the catheter. The catheter should be inserted up to this point with the markers on the catheter. The catheter should be inserted up to this point when it is placed; for heavy individuals, 1 or 3 additional cm may be required to allow for the distance between the skin and the vein (Fig. 3.1).
- Open catheter tray in sterile fashion and keep in easy reach.
- Uncap distal catheter lumen only, prepare the J-wire, draw 1% lidocaine into a syringe and place 4 × 4 gauze pads in easy reach.

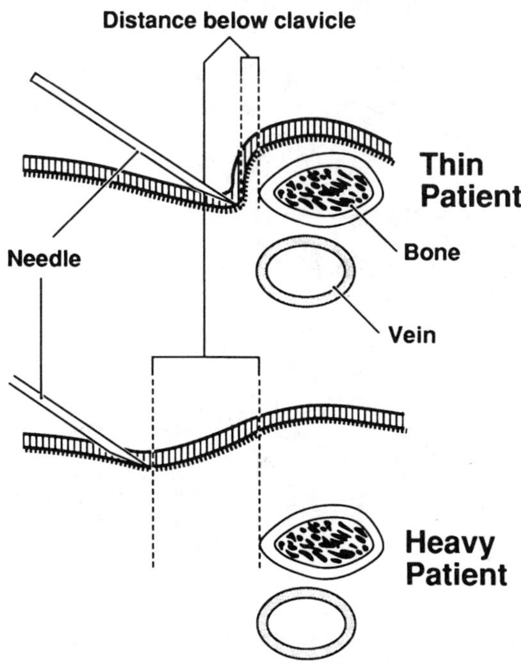

Figure 3.2.
Distance below clavicle.

- Position needle snugly on syringe so that the bevel markings are opposite the syringe markings for easy viewing. The needle should be easy to remove so that it is not dislodged from the vein when the needle is removed after cannulation.
- Infiltrate skin at site of cannulation with 1% lidocaine using a 22 gauge needle. This needle may also be used as a "finder" needle for the vein itself. The needle should be inserted to the clavicle with lidocaine injected into the periosteum. Do not advance the needle unless the syringe is aspirated so that an arterial or venous puncture can be detected immediately.
- Keep the needle parallel to the floor and angled up toward the sternal notch, and lidocaine can be injected as the needle is slowly removed.
- Cannulate the vein at the clavicular angle (junction of the medial ⅓ and lateral ⅔). The skin will be penetrated very near the point where the vein is cannulated in thin or cachexic patients. In heavier individuals, the skin should be penetrated more inferior and slightly more lateral to allow an angle of attack to permit entry from under the clavicle into the vein (Fig. 3.3).
- The cannulating needle should then be inserted through the anesthetized tract, contact made with the anesthetized portion of the clavicle, and the needle "walked" under the clavicle along the same path as the "finder" needle. Always aspirate the needle while advancing until venous blood is returned. If no blood can be aspirated, the needle should be slowly withdrawn while aspirating because the vein may have been penetrated in a through-

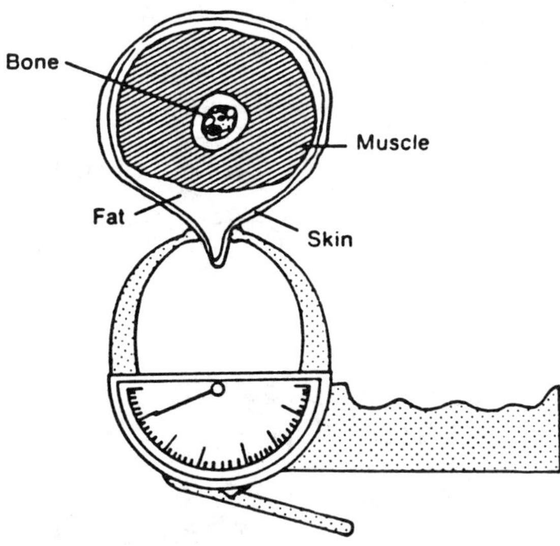

Figure 3.3.
This cross-section shows the technique for measuring a skinfold, a double layer of subcutaneous fat and skin. In this case, the triceps skinfold is being measured with the Lang caliper. (Reprinted with permission from Grant, A. Nutritional Assessment Guidelines. Berkeley, California, Cutter Laboratories, 1979.)

and-through manner. The lumen may be entered while withdrawing the needle.

- Stabilize the needle against the chest wall and remove the syringe once the vein has been cannulated.
- Advance the J-wire through the needle and into the vein.
- If resistance is encountered, withdraw the wire slowly and try again. If resistance to withdrawing the wire occurs, remove both wire and needle to avoid shearing off the end of the wire with the subsequent distal embolization.
- Withdraw the needle after half of the wire has been passed into the vein.
- Incise the skin at the site of entrance of the wire with a #11 blade (in kit) over the wire and into the vein. Twisting the dilator while advancing may help. Do not advance the wire with the dilator. Failure to pass the dilator may indicate a bent wire.
- Withdraw the dilator once it has been passed into the vein and apply pressure to the skin site to prevent bleeding.
- Insert the catheter over the guidewire until the wire emerges from the distal port. Grasp the wire and advance the catheter into the vein to the previously measured point.
- Remove the wire. Attach a syringe to the distal port to prevent venous air embolism.
- Flush the ports and fix the catheter to the skin with suture (Fig. 3.4) and apply sterile dressing.
- Perform a chest radiograph to ascertain correct placement. If PN is being considered for a period of more than 2 weeks, a Hickman or similar cuffed, tunneled catheter is placed to reduce the risk of line sepsis. A PICC may also be appropriate.

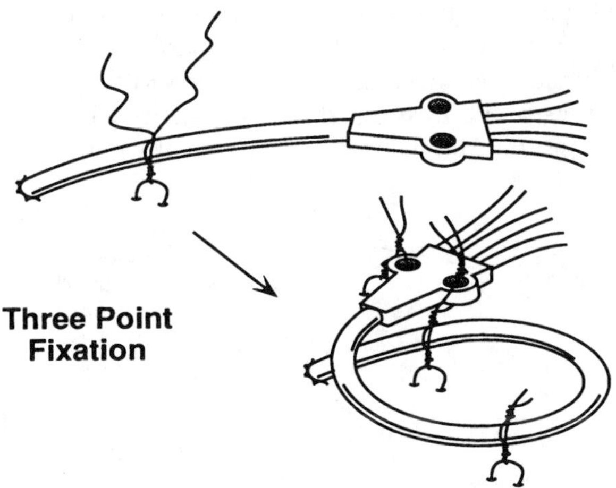

Figure 3.4.
Three point fixation.

Hickman, Broviac or Groshong Catheter Placement

- Technique is the same as for a triple lumen catheter except that it is placed in the operating room where sterility is better controlled and additional sedation may be used if necessary.
- Two small skin incisions are necessary about 5–7 cm apart. The cuff should be placed just beneath the skin surface of the lower incision for easy removal under local anesthesia at a later date if necessary. The catheter should be well secured (Fig. 3.5). It usually takes approximately 3–4 weeks for fibrous tissue to grow through the cuff. Therefore, the securing suture can be removed after that time if it is irritating for the patient.
- Proper tip placement in the vena cava should be verified by radiograph. A C-arm fluoroscope is unnecessary, costly, exposes the patient and personnel to additional radiation and may be inferior to chest radiograph for determining proper catheter placement.

Catheter Care and Use Protocol (Adapted from UCLA Nursing Care Protocols)

Site Care (All Catheters)

1. Clean catheter exit site with (3) alcohol saturated applicators, followed by (3) povidone-iodine saturated applicators using the following principles:
   a. Apply in circular motion at site and work from center outward; do not re-use the same applicator over a previously cleaned area.
   b. Use single use applicator, then discard; and use some type of applicator to avoid hand contamination.
   c. Excess solution is not wiped off—let povidone-iodine dry. Wet povidone-iodine is *not* bactericidal.
2. Apply povidone-iodine ointment to the catheter exit site.
   a. Dress with gauze or sterile transparent dressing. Gauze dressings should be changed daily or every other day; more often if saturated. Transparent dressings should be changed 1–3 times weekly. Dressings should be changed more frequently in neutropenic patients.

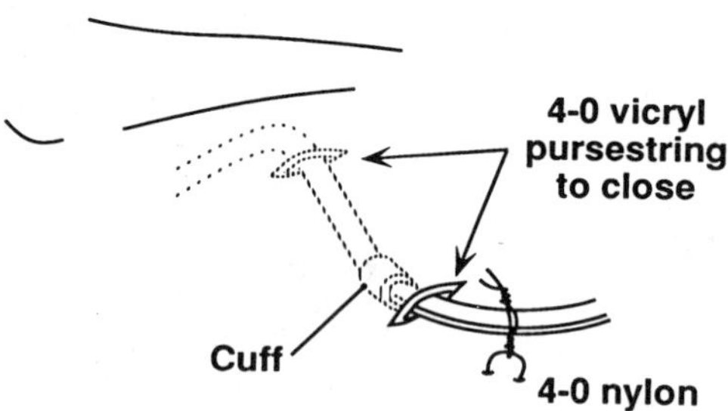

Figure 3.5.
4–0 pursestring to close.

HUB Care

HUB Care: Short-term CVCs	Hub Care: Long-TermCVCs
Scrub with **povidone-iodine** for 30 seconds prior to opening	Scrub junction with (3) **alcohol** Scrub junction with (3) **povidone-iodine** Open port

* The hub may be a common source for catheter infection.

CVC Hub Care

CVC hub care should be done before any opening of the CVC at the level of the hub and **prior to** removal of CVC cap or cap change or CVC tubing change or tubing discontinuation.

Long-Term CVC Hub Care Procedure. (Tunneled silastic, PICC lines, subcutaneous infusion ports)

1. Clean work surface with alcohol and wash hands thoroughly.
2. Set up supplies
   (3) applicators saturated in alcohol
   (3) applicators saturated in povidone-iodine
   (2) alcohol prep pads
   CVC occlusion forceps if no reattached clamps on line
   2-inch plastic tape
3. Use clean, non-sterile gloves if contact with blood or secretions is anticipated and remove tape at junction of the CVC hub and cap/IV tubing.
4. Scrub from catheter junction site outward in a circular manner first using alcohol saturated applicators, then povidone-iodine saturated applicators. Extend cleansed area approximately 2 inches on either side of the junction, then clamp CVC.
5. With alcohol prep wrapped around both sides of the junction, remove CVC cap or IV tubing. Continue to hold CVC with first alcohol wipe and perform necessary CVC care (cap change, tubing change, blood draw, heparin flush).
6. Replace CVC cap or IV tubing as necessary. Tape the junction securely with 2-inch plastic tape.

Short-Term CVC Hub Care Procedure. (Triple, double, single lumen, Cordis, Swan-Ganz, arterial lines)
Scrub hub with **povidone-iodine** for 30 seconds.

Injection Port Care

Scrub with **povidone-iodine** 30 seconds before accessing port.

CVC Injection Port Care

CVC port care should be done before any entry of any injection port on the CVC or on IV lines connected to the CVC This includes the following:

a. Injection cap ports
b. Buretrol injection ports (not usually used with PN lines)
c. Injection ports on IV lines connected to CVCs

Long-Term CVC Port Care Procedure. (Tunneled or short-term silastic, PICC lines, subcutaneous infusion ports)

Wash hands thoroughly. Use clean nonsterile gloves if contact with blood or secretions is anticipated, and scrub injection port vigorously with povidone-iodine for 30 seconds.

IV Tubing Change

1. *All* IV tubing on *all* lines should be changed every 72 hours, EXCEPT for: TPN sets (amino acid/dextrose and intralipid solutions), which should be changed daily.
2. Portable CADD and PCA units: tubing should be changed with cassette changes.
3. Stopcocks, y-connectors, and extension sets should be changed with tubing changes.

CVC Care Principles

1. All procedures for CVC care are designed to prevent infections and mechanical complications of use. Aseptic technique should be maintained in all handling of the CVC and all attached lines.
2. Universal precautions should be observed at all times in handling the CVC.
3. For infusion in non-emergent situations after CVC placement, placement of catheter tip should be confirmed radiologically before it can be used for infusion.
4. The CVC multi-stick injection cap should be changed every week even if the catheter is not in use.
5. An infusion control device should always be used to administer primary IV fluids via the CVC to prevent blood backup and clot formation in the line.

CVC Dressing Care

The CVC exit site may be dressed with either:

1. Sterile gauze and tape—change daily or every other day.

   or

2. Sterile transparent dressing—change 1–3 times weekly.

The nurse may decide which type of dressing best meets the individual patient's needs. Patients who may not tolerate a sterile transparent dressing include:

1. Diaphoretic patients.
2. Patients with fragile skin (irradiated skin) or drainage at the CVC site.
3. Neutropenic patients.
4. Patient's preference should also be considered when dealing with patients with established CVCs.

Patients may develop irritation of the skin at the CVC site in response to the various cleansing agents used. Substitutions in cleansing agents may be made according to patient needs or preference.

Patients with Hickman, Broviac or Groshong-type catheters that have been in place more than 2–3 weeks may shower or bathe. After shower, wet dressing is removed, skin is cleansed per protocol and redressed. If showering prior to this, the exit site and catheter should be covered with a water tight dressing.

CVC Dressing Change Procedure

a. Disinfect work area with alcohol and wash hands thoroughly.
b. Set up supplies:
    1. (3) applicators saturated in alcohol
    2. (3) applicators saturated in povidone-iodine
    3. Povidone-iodine ointment
    4. Dressing—2 × 2 sterile gauze pad and tape or sterile transparent dressing
c. Have patient turn head away and remove old dressing. Look for erythema, drainage or signs of catheter dislodgement at exit site.
d. Clean from exit site outward in circular motion, first using alcohol saturated applicator, then povidone-iodine saturated applicators, cleansing an area of approximately 2 inches in diameter.
e. Apply small amount (pea-sized drop) of povidone-iodine ointment at exit site.
f. Apply dressing and secure the CVC to prevent dislodgement.

Percutaneously Inserted Central Catheters (PICC) Line Dressing Guidelines

a. When removing old dressing, pull it off toward the shoulder to avoid dislodging catheter (in most cases, steri-strips will be used to secure the catheter in place). Alternatively, the PICC may be anchored to the skin using a suture. Cleansing may be done over/around the strips (if strips are intact). Strips **must be changed weekly.**
b. Newly placed PICC lines may require pressure dressing for the first 24 hours to prevent bleeding or hematoma formation. After this time, a transparent or gauze dressing should be placed. If insertion was diffi-

cult and the vein traumatized, a prophylactic heating pad used for 20 minutes every 6 hours over the next 24 hours may help prevent phlebitis.

c. The site may be covered with Kerlix® if patient objects to the site of the PICC.

Heparin Flush Guidelines

Heparin flush is unnecessary for continuous infusions.

Heparin Flush Dosing: Standard heparin flush: 3 ml of 100 units/ml heparin (300 units) per lumen of CVC.

Pediatrics (and small adults): 50 units/kg body weight maximum per day—(per *day,* not per flush, or per lumen)

CVCs should be heparin flushed under the following circumstances:

1. When capped (not in use for continuous infusion): every 24 hours. (Exception: Pediatric Arrowcath®, flush q 4–6 hr when capped).
2. When discontinuing IV infusions, after administration of intermittent IV medications or fluids.
3. After CVC blood draws, as needed.
4. PICC Lines: 1.5 ml of 100 units/ml heparin (150 units)
5. Subcutaneous infusion ports: Standard heparin flush: 5 ml of 100 units/ml heparin (500 units) plus 5 ml of 0.9% sodium chloride. See Appendix 1, Table 18—CVC care chart for other flushing guidelines.
6. Groshong CVC: Use 5 ml 0.9% sodium chloride for flushing. See Appendix 1, Table 18—CVC care chart for other flushing guidelines.

Blood Drawing Via CVC

If coagulation studies are obtained through the CVC, it is necessary to aspirate 6 ml of blood before drawing samples for coagulation studies. Label requisition slip, "Drawn from __________ line."

The CVC may be used for drawing of blood cultures. The discard specimen may also be used for blood cultures.

Blood Drawing Via CVC Syringe Method

1. Determine amount of blood needed for tests ordered. Collect appropriate tubes and supplies; use clean, nonsterile gloves. Cleanse CVC hub using appropriate CVC hub care procedure and clamp all lumens of CVC. Lumens that are not being used for blood draw should remain clamped throughout procedure.
   NOTE: The following steps must be done quickly so that the line does not clog.
2. Attach sterile syringe to CVC. Unclamp CVC and withdraw 6 ml of blood for discard unless the aspirated blood is to be returned, then clamp CVC and attach another sterile syringe.

3. Unclamp CVC and aspirate blood specimen. Continue steps 7 and 8 until all specimens are obtained, using a new sterile syringe each time. After appropriate specimens have been obtained, clamp CVC. The original aspirate may be returned at this time.
4. Flush CVC with 3–5 ml of 0.9% sodium chloride as necessary, followed by appropriate heparin flush. Recap the CVC or attach IV tubing to continue infusion and inject aspirated blood into appropriate tubes.

If needling through injection port to perform syringe blood draw:

1. Attach 20 gauge needles to blood draw syringes.
2. Cleanse injection port according to CVC injection port care procedure, before beginning procedure.

Vacutainer® CVC Blood Draw Procedure.

1. Determine amount of blood needed for tests. Collect appropriate tubes and supplies and a 7 ml red top blood collection tube for discard or clot for the blood bank if necessary.
2. Attach vacutainer and vacutainer Luer adaptor together (it is unnecessary to remove rubber cover of needle end inserted into vacutainer), and use clean, unsterile gloves.
3. Clean CVC hub using appropriate hub care procedure.
4. Stop infusion and clamp all lumens of CVC and disconnect IV tubing or cap on lumen to be used for blood draw.
5. Attach vacutainer to central line hub and unclamp CVC on blood draw lumen only and draw 7 ml for discard (use 7 ml red top tube), then attach other blood specimen tubes to vacutainer to obtain ordered specimens (draw coagulation studies last). Clamp CVC after blood specimens are drawn and remove vacutainer.
6. Flush CVC with 3–5 ml of 0.9% sodium chloride as necessary, followed by appropriate heparin flush. Recap CVC or attach IV tubing to continue infusion.
   Vacutainer holder is placed in plastic specimen cup containing alcohol (cover all of holder with alcohol).

If needling through injection cap to perform vacutainer blood draw:

1. Attach a 20 gauge needle, 1″ long or less, into the Luer lock adaptor of the vacutainer holder.
2. Clean injection cap using CVC injection port care procedure.

Assessing Subcutaneous Infusion Ports (Port-a-caths®)

Subcutaneous infusion ports may be accessed using a Huber needle for intermittent or continuous administration of IV fluids or medications.

1. Clean work surface with alcohol and wash hands thoroughly.
2. Assemble supplies:
   (3) applicators saturated with alcohol
   (3) applicators saturated with povidone-iodine
   (1) pair sterile gloves
   (1) Huber needle ("Gripper" or standard)
   Gripper needle comes with extension set attached. If using standard Huber, attach microbore extension tubing to needle.
   (1) 5-ml syringe filled with 0.9% sodium chloride solution
3. Palpate port site to locate portal septum.
4. Clean area over port site with (3) alcohol saturated applicators, followed by (3) povidone-iodine saturated applicators. With each applicator, start at the center of the port site and work outward in a circular motion to cover an area approximately 4 inches in diameter. Use sterile gloves.
5. Connect 5-ml syringe with sodium chloride to extension tubing on Huber needle and purge extension tubing and needle. *Maintaining sterility of the Huber needle is essential.*
6. Locate portal septum by palpation and insert Huber needle perpendicular to the septum, pushing it firmly through the skin and portal septum until it hits the bottom of the portal chamber.
7. Slowly inject approximately 3 ml of 0.9% sodium chloride into port, noting any resistance. Aspirate solution to check for blood return. If bubbling is observed around the needle when flushing, port may not be accessed properly. Remove needle and attempt to reaccess port.
8. Slowly inject remainder of sodium chloride and clamp extension set and remove syringe, then attach appropriate IV tubing and administer solutions/medications as ordered.

Huber needle should be changed weekly when left in place for continuous infusion. Change dressing over port weekly.

Extension sets may be capped with multi-stick caps, and the port may be used for intermittent administration of IV fluids and medications. The port must be flushed daily and after each intermittent infusion under these circumstances. To remove Huber needle from port:

1. Clean work surfaces with alcohol and wash hands thoroughly.
2. Prepare supplies:
   (1) 20 ml syringe filled with 5 ml of 100 units/ml heparin (500 units) and 5 ml 0.9% sodium chloride.
   Clean, non-sterile gloves
3. Clamp extension tubing on Huber needle, clean junction, and disconnect IV tubing.
4. Attach 10-ml syringe with heparin and saline to extension tubing and unclamp extension tubing and slowly inject approximately 8 ml of heparin-sodium chloride solution into port.
5. Withdraw Huber needle by maintaining positive pressure on syringe while simultaneously withdrawing the needle and pressing down

on the port with two fingers. This will prevent reflux of blood into port.

Home Care

Patients requiring long-term central venous access may be discharged home with their CVC. It is not advisable to discharge patients with temporary-access CVCs, such as percutaneous Cook® and Arrow® catheters. All other types of CVCs may be considered safe for home use.

It is recommended that teaching for patients going home with a capped CVC begin at least 3 days before anticipated date of discharge. Ideally, patient teaching should begin as soon as it is known that the line will be placed. If the patient cannot care for the line, a family member or significant other should be identified to learn the necessary care procedures. *The patient and/or significant other should receive instruction in the following:*

1. CVC dressing change
2. Heparin flush of the CVC via injection cap
3. CVC injection cap change
4. Home problem solving and follow-up care

It is helpful to provide the patient with written instructions accompanied by diagrams.

COMPONENTS OF PARENTERAL NUTRITION SOLUTIONS

Fluid Volume

In a fluid-restricted patient, both dextrose and amino acid concentrations can be increased. A higher proportion of calories may also be supplied using lipid emulsion, which is more calorically dense than dextrose (see section on lipid emulsion). See section regarding fluid requirements.

Dextrose

a. Because it is more cost-effective to use "standard" TPN formulations, 25% dextrose (monohydrate) (250 g/l) is most often used = 3.4 kcal/ml (example: 1 liter D25 provides 850 kcal).
b. The maximum dextrose concentration that can be peripherally infused is 10% (with no more than 3.5% amino acids). The maximum osmolality of peripherally administered fluids should be ≤ 900 mOsm. Therefore, in average to large sized individuals, it is nearly impossible to supply their entire caloric requirement via the peripheral route. The maximum dextrose concentration that should be centrally infused is 35%. See Appendix 1, Table 19 for osmolalities of parenteral nutrients.
c. The minimum dextrose requirement is approximately 200 g daily, primarily for the brain.

d. The maximum glucose oxidation rate is 7 mg/kg/min (7).
e. For patients receiving CAPD, the amount of glucose absorption from the dialysate should be estimated and included in the calculation of delivered calories.

Dialysis Solutions
1.5% = 1.3 g/dL glucose
2.5% = 2.2 g/L glucose
4.25% = 3.76 g/L glucose

Absorbed glucose (g) = [11.3 (glucose conc. in dialysate) − 10.9] × volume of exchanges
Absorbed calories = glucose (g) × 3.7 kcal/kg
(Approximately 60–80% of glucose is absorbed)

Protein (Amino Acids)

Standard Formulations

Crystalline amino acids are available in standard concentrations of 8.5–15%, although other concentrations can be provided for the proper indications. The amino acid solution is diluted with an appropriate amount of dextrose to achieve a desired concentration, usually 3.5–5.0%. These include a final concentration of < 3.5% in non-oliguric renal and/or hepatic failure (in the absence of dialysis) or a final concentration of > 4.25% in fluid restriction (see Appendix 1, Tables 20–22 for protein supply and for the amino acid formulation of parenteral nutrition solutions).

Some amino acid formulas may contain sodium bisulfite as a preservative. Patients with hypersensitivity to sulfa should not receive these formulas.

Specialty Formulations

- High cost when compared with standard amino acid solutions.
- See Appendix 1, Table 23 for the various specialty formulations available and their amino acid components.

Hepatic Disease (HepatAmine®)

- High in branched chain amino acids.
- Low in aromatic amino acids.
- May be useful in patients with hepatic encephalopathy (Grade II or greater or with chronic hepatic encephalopathy) who otherwise would be unable to tolerate sufficient standard amino acid infusion. If encephalopathy is secondary to sepsis, gastrointestinal hemorrhage, uremia or electrolyte imbalance, there is no role for HepatAmine®. For further discussion, see *branched chain amino acids.*

Renal

See discussion on parenteral formulas.

High Branched Chain

See discussion on parenteral formulas.

Lipid Emulsion

- Lipid emulsions are isotonic and may be infused via peripheral vein. They are an especially valuable caloric source if peripheral parenteral nutrition is used.
- Used for a caloric source (typically 20–30% of total calories and to prevent essential fatty acid deficiency).
- 10% emulsion provides 1.1 kcal/ml and the 20% emulsion provides 2.0 kcal/ml (for comparison, D25 provides 0.85 kcal/ml and D35 1.1 kcal/ml) (see Appendix 1, Tables 24 and 25 for caloric supply composition of lipid emulsions)
- A test dose of 0.5 ml/min over 15–30 min for 20% emulsion, or 1 ml/min for 10% emulsion is recommended to test emulsion stability and hypersensitivity.
- Maximum infusion rate is 100 ml/hr for the 10% emulsion and 50 ml/hr for the 20% emulsion to prevent overload of the reticular endothelial system.
- Maximum total infusion is 2.5 g/kg/day to avoid "fat overload syndrome" which is characterized by hepatomegaly, jaundice, thrombocytopenia, and death.
- Maximum hang time for any bottle of lipid emulsion is 12 hours. There is evidence that 3:1 solution may be safely hung longer.
- Should not be used in patients who have allergy to eggs. Rare instances of anaphylaxis have been reported. Egg phosphatides are used as emulsifying agents.
- Uncommon side effects include fever, headache, back pain, dyspnea, chills, nausea, chest pain, and oily taste.
- May be used in pancreatitis not associated with hypertriglyceridemia as long as serum triglyceride concentration is monitored as with any other patient receiving intravenous lipids.
- No evidence in humans that the use of lipid emulsion induces premature labor.
- Soybean allergy is <u>not</u> a contraindication as the emulsion contains no soy protein.
- Triglyceride level should be checked 4–6 hours after the infusion has ceased to ascertain adequate clearance.
- Can be administered in a "piggyback" form with parenteral nutrition solutions via an injection port or administered directly. Lipid emulsion is also a constituent of 3 in 1 solutions (dextrose, lipid, amino acids).
- Lipids are not routinely administered through a filter unless 3 in 1 mixtures are used. In this situation, a 1.2 micron filter should be used to exclude particulate matter; bacteria will not be excluded. Filter pore size $<$ 1.2 micron will not permit lipid to pass.

Essential Fatty Acid Deficiency

Need minimum of 2–4% of total calories as linoleic acid for prevention (lipid emulsion is 50% linoleic acid).

Electrolytes

- Parenteral electrolyte content must be adjusted according to serum electrolyte concentration.
- Electrolyte imbalances should be corrected if possible before initiating PN.
- PN should not be used as replacement fluid for additional losses beyond maintenance.
- Sodium bicarbonate interferes with calcium-phosphate compatibility and should be avoided in parenteral nutrition solutions. Acetate salt should be used as a bicarbonate substitute. Sodium bicarbonate should never be injected through a catheter used for parenteral nutrition.
- To avoid alkalosis or hyperchloremic metabolic acidosis, the chloride to sodium ratio should be 1:1.

Acetate and Chloride

The pharmacist will balance the concentration of acetate and chloride in parenteral nutrition solutions to prevent hyperchloremic metabolic acidosis or hypochloremic metabolic alkalosis. In hyperchloremic metabolic acidosis, the acetate concentration can be maximized. This requires the addition of sodium and potassium (as acetate salts). The other option is to minimize the chloride concentration. This may be the only option if additional sodium and potassium cannot be added to the parenteral nutrition solution. Before manipulating the parenteral nutrition solution, attempt to correct any underlying disorder such as vomiting, diarrhea, or nasogastric suction losses.

Phosphate

Phosphate is provided in parenteral nutrition solutions as either a sodium or a potassium salt. Therefore, when the phosphate concentration is increased from the standard, the sodium and/or potassium concentration should be correspondingly increased when possible. However, phosphate is ordered in *mmol,* not mEq, and is *not* in 1:1 ratio with the sodium or potassium salt (Tables 3.1 and 3.2).

Calcium-Phosphate Solubility

The most commonly encountered compatibility problem encountered in parenteral nutrition solutions is the addition of calcium and phosphate. Precipita-

Table 3.1.
Parenteral Phosphate Products

	Phosphate	Sodium	Potassium
Sodium phosphate	3 mmol	4 mEq	0
Potassium phosphate	3 mmol	–	4.4 mEq

Table 3.2.
Phosphate Conversion

mmol PO_4	ml added	mEq Na	mEq K
3	1.0	4	4.4
4	1.3	5	5.7
5	1.7	7	7.5
6	2.0	8	8.8
7	2.3	9	9.7
8	2.7	11	11.9
9	3.0	12	13.2
10	3.3	13	14.5

tion may occur in the form of dibasic calcium phosphate crystals. These crystals may be apparent in the solution or become apparent only when the PN catheter lumen becomes occluded.

Calcium-phosphate solubility is dependent on several factors:

1. Relative molar Ca and P concentrations
2. Amino acid formula and concentration (the lower the concentration, the less soluble Ca-P)
3. Dextrose concentration (the lower the concentration, the less soluble Ca-P)
4. Temperature (less soluble at higher temperature)
5. pH of PN solution (dibasic precipitates form at high pH)
6. Order of compounding of the solution (Ca should be added last)

These variables make it difficult to set a maximum calcium or phosphate concentration. As a guideline, a maximum phosphate concentration of 17 mmol/L can be achieved with any solution containing calcium ≤ 5 mEq/L. Phosphate concentration should never exceed 25 mmol/L even in solutions of high dextrose and amino acid concentration. Extraordinary calcium or phosphate losses should be replaced separately from PN (Fig. 3.6).
Consult the pharmacy when additional calcium or phosphate are necessary.

Vitamins and Minerals

- One vial of multivitamins should be provided daily in the first liter of parenteral nutrition solution.
- The vitamin concentrations in this formulation are based on the recommendations of the AMA Nutritional Advisory Group (1979) (see Appendix 1, Table 26).
- If the patient receives less than 1 liter of PN in a 24-hour period, the volume of vitamin and mineral infusion should be increased proportionately or one vial of multivitamins in 100 ml of D5W or 0.9% NaCl should be administered over 2 hours.

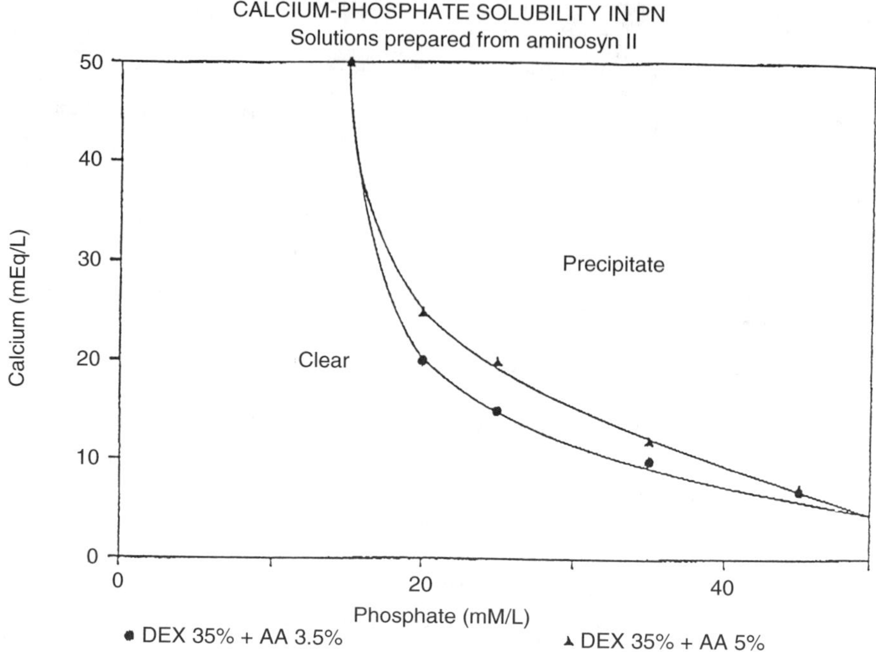

Figure 3.6.
Calcium-phosphate solubility in PN. (Reprinted with permission from Abbott Labs, North Chicago, IL.)

- The multivitamin formula does not include vitamin K (phytonadione). However, 1 mg of vitamin K may be added daily to PN solution by the pharmacy on a routine basis unless otherwise ordered. Therefore, the prothrombin time (PT) would not require weekly monitoring. Patients who are to be anticoagulated should not receive vitamin K.
- Long-term use of vitamin A should be avoided in renal failure because of the possibility of toxic accumulation as it is not removed during dialysis. Serum vitamin D and E levels should be monitored during renal failure (see Appendix 1, Table 17 for information on signs of vitamin deficiency).

Iron

- Not routinely supplied in parenteral nutrition solutions, therefore, intravenous iron dextran (Imferon®) supplementation may be necessary. Iron dextran may not be available to the bone marrow.
- The dose may be calculated using the equation:

$$0.66 \times \text{body wt [kg]} \times \frac{(100 - \text{Hgb (g/dl)} \times 100)}{14\text{g}}$$

For example, in an adult patient with a Hgb of 8.2 g/L weighing 68 kg:

$$\text{Iron deficit} = 0.66 \times 68 \times \frac{(100 - 8.2 \times 100)}{14.8} = 2925 \text{ mg}$$

Total amount of iron dextran necessary:

$$\frac{2925 \text{ mg}}{50 \text{ mg/ml}} = 58.5 \text{ ml}$$

This may be infused in daily doses of 2 mL (100 mg—the maximum for 29 consecutive days). The maximum dose is 100 mg daily because larger doses have been associated with severe arthralgias and paralysis (manufacturers' guidelines).

Before beginning iron dextran replacement, a free flowing IV is started and a "test dose" of 25 mg in 100 ml of 0.9 NaCl is administered over 1–2 hours. The vein should be flushed with normal saline after the infusion is completed. Epinephrine (0.3 ml of 1:1000 solution) should be available at the bedside should anaphylaxis occur. Alternatively, iron dextran may be added to parenteral nutrition solutions although the pharmacy should be contacted should non-standard additives be present in the solution because of limited compatibility data.

Trace Elements

- One vial of multi-trace elements (zinc, chromium, manganese, copper, selenium) should be provided daily in the first liter of parenteral nutrition. Chromium supplementation may be unnecessary, but it is currently included in the multiple formulation.
- Copper should be withheld in cases of severe cholestasis.
- Selenium requirement may increase in renal failure.
- See Appendix 1, Table 16 for signs of trace element deficiency.
- Sufficient iodine is supplied via povidone-iodine use and subsequent absorption through the skin.
- Nickel, molybdenum, vanadium, tin, silicon, fluoride, arsenic may be required trace elements, but their necessity has been only demonstrated in animals.

Additives

Insulin

- If a patient's blood sugar is sufficiently elevated as to require a continuous insulin drip, PN should not be initiated until glucose is controlled. The blood glucose should be < 200 mg/dL before PN is started.
- May be necessary to control glucose intolerance.
- When insulin is necessary, usually one unit of <u>regular</u> insulin per 10 g dextrose (e.g., 10 units with D10, 25 units with D25) will be sufficient. This should be added directly to the parenteral nutrition solution during compounding. The suggested maximum insulin should be 2.0 units regular insulin per gram of dextrose (i.e., 50 units/l of D25). If hyperglycemia con-

tinues, the dextrose concentration should be reduced and the source for the hyperglycemia investigated.

- A sliding scale should be ordered to cover hyperglycemic episodes despite the addition of insulin to the parenteral nutrition solution. However, the addition of a corresponding amount of insulin should be added to the parenteral nutrition solution of subsequently compounded bottles. No insulin or additional dextrose should be added to the bottle during the infusion as this violates the closed system and increases the risk of infection.
- If additional insulin is necessary, add ⅔ of the previous day's sliding scale dosage to the PN. Make certain to divide the total insulin dose by the number of liters of PN daily.
- The patient's glucose should be kept below 200 mg/dL to avoid glucosuria with subsequent fluid and electrolyte loss and during infections, impaired neutrophil chemotaxis and NK ability. However, because of the risk of overshooting and causing hypoglycemia, control below 120–140 mg/dL is undesirable except during pregnancy when the blood sugar should be < 120 mg/dL.
- Insulin adsorbs to both glass and plastic bottles and tubing and this factor, though small, should be considered when determining insulin dosage, especially in highly sensitive diabetic patients.
- A sliding scale or separate continuous intravenous insulin infusion should always be used when insulin requirements are unstable to avoid the wastage of PN.
- Increased plasma insulin activates the Na-K ATPase pump, which shifts potassium intracellularly and decreases serum potassium concentration.

Heparin, Hydrocortisone

One thousand units of heparin and 5–10 mg hydrocortisone may be added to each liter of peripheral parenteral nutrition because evidence suggests a decrease in the risk of phlebitis (2, 8).

Albumin

The use of albumin infusions in nutrition support is controversial. What is not controversial, however, is the fact that exogenous albumin infusion will **not** directly improve a patient's nutritional status. Albumin infusion, if used at all, should only be used specifically to improve plasma oncotic pressure and treat hypo-oncotic edema (9). Albumin provides up to 75% of the normal oncotic pressure in the intravascular space especially when the serum concentration is < 3.0 g/dL (10). However, there is little increase in the oncotic pressure as the serum albumin increases above 3.0 g/dL (11). It remains unclear if the provision of exogenous albumin leads to improved enteral formula tolerance in hypoalbuminemic patients. One study showed an improvement when serum albumin was increased from 3.0 to 3.4 g/dL (12) and another found that patients with a capillary oncotic pressure < 18 mm Hg had enteral feeding intolerance while those with a COP > 18 mm Hg did not (13). Other studies have found that enteral feeding tolerance was unaffected by the serum albumin concentration and 97% of patients with an albumin < 2.5 g/dL tolerated enteral feeding (14, 15). An area that has not been addressed in albumin infusion studies is the effect of albumin infusion on mitigating medication side effects due to alteration in drug delivery and elimination related to hypoalbuminemia.

If the use of albumin supplementation is contemplated, a slow infusion should be used rather than rapid bolus injection as the half-life is prolonged in the former and increased serum albumin concentration may persist for up to a week (16). The total albumin deficit should be calculated and used as an end-point in the use of supplemental albumin:

$$\text{Deficit (g)} = \text{weight(kg)} \times 3\ \text{dL/kg} \times 3.5 - \text{initial serum albumin g/dL}$$

where the 3 dL/kg reflects the average percent of exchangeable albumin in the plasma compartment (16).

H_2 Antagonists

H_2 antagonists may be added to parenteral nutrition solutions to control excessive gastric secretion in new onset short bowel syndrome, stress ulcer prophylaxis, or treatment of peptic ulcer disease. In fact, it is more cost-effective to add these medications to the parenteral nutrition solutions than to hang separate infusions.

Antibiotics

Typically, antibiotics are not added to parenteral nutrition solutions. However, consult Appendix 1, Tables 28 and 29 for compatibility of the TPN line to be used for the antibiotic infusion. The use of a dedicated TPN line for additional infusions is discouraged if alternate infusion sites are available, unless catheter infection is being treated.

WRITING ORDERS

Parenteral Nutrition Order Form

- All orders for parenteral nutrition should be written on a parenteral nutrition order form so that all necessary ingredients can be easily ordered in their appropriate concentrations.
- Orders to initiate TPN should contain indication, height, and weight. This is helpful for quality control and for basic nutritional assessment.
- Any changes to the parenteral nutrition solution require the entire solution formula to be rewritten unless only the rate is changed. That way, the current PN formulation can be obtained from the patient record on an immediate basis if necessary, both in case of emergency and to save time by avoiding the need to search through the chart. If only the rate is changed, the Parenteral Nutrition Order Form should still be used, but only the new rate indicated and the form clearly marked "rate change only." (See sample Parenteral Nutrition Order Form, Fig. 3.7)

Adult Parenteral Nutrition Solution Orders
Baylor College of Medicine 6550 Fannin, Houston, TX 77030
Use BallPoint Pen - Press Firmly

Check Box:
☐ **Initiation Orders** ☐ **Change of Therapy** ☐ **Rate change only** ☐ **Discontinuation**
PN orders will not be filled by the pharmacy in the absence of indication and estimated needs unless rate change only. When change of therapy is checked, all PN solutions already made will be used unless otherwise ordered.

CONSULTS	Check Box: ☐ NST Clerk: Please notify
INDICATION FOR TPN	
ESTIMATED NEEDS	**Height** ___ inches **Current Weight** ___ kg **Ideal Body Weight** ___ kg Estimated caloric requirement ________ kcal/day (25-35 kcal/kg/day for maintenance, 40 kcal/kg/day for repletion) Estimated protein requirement ________ g/day (1.0-1.5 g/kg/day)* *May not be appropriate in hepatic or renal failure ☐ **Check box** to order **Indirect Calorimetry** to estimate resting energy expenditure and to determine caloric requirement.
FORMULA	**CHECK BOX FOR DESIRED FORMULA:**

1. PERIPHERAL **CENTRAL**
☐ Dextrose 10%-Amino Acid 3.5% ☐ Dextrose 25%-Amino Acid 4.25% ☐ OTHER ____________
(340 non-protein kcal/L) (35 g protein/L) (850 g/L non-protein kcal/L) (42.5 g protein/L)

2. ELECTROLYTES Check one:

☐ **Standard Electrolytes**		☐ **Custom Electrolytes** (Write as totals per L)		**Chloride and Acetate**
Na 35 mEq/L		Na _____ mEq/L		☐ Minimize Cl, max. Ac (for acidosis)
K 30 mEq/L	Mg 10 mEq/L	K _____ mEq/L	Mg ____ mEq/L	☐ Max. Cl, minimize Ac (for alkalosis)
Ca 5 mEq/L	P 10 mMol/L	Ca _____ mEq/L	P ____ mMol/L	☐ Balance CL & Ac
				☐ Ac _____ Cl _____

3. VITAMINS AND TRACE ELEMENTS
Unless otherwise ordered, MVI-12, Vitamin K_1 mg/day, and Multi-trace elements (Zn 3mg, Cr 12µg, Cu 1.2mg, Se 40µg, Mn 0.3mg) will be included in each daily TPN solution. Additional supplementation should be ordered under "Other".

4. ADDITIVES
Regular Human Insulin ______ U/L H_2 Blocker ______________ mg/24hrs Other______________

5. LIPID EMULSION Check Box
☐ 10% 500 ml (1.1 kcal/mL) ☐ 20% 200 ml (2.0 kcal/mL) ☐ 20% 500 ml (2.0 kcal/mL) Frequency_____

RATE	**Check one box and fill in blanks:** ☐ Start central PN at ___ mL/hr for ___ hrs, increase to ___ mL/hr for ____ hrs, then increase to ____ mL/hr thereafter (goal) ☐ Infuse at ____ mL/hr **All fat emulsion infused at 50 mL/hr**
MONITORING	Nursing • Daily weights, strict inputs and outputs, temperature every 8 hours • Accucheck 2 hrs after every rate increase, then q.6h x 3 days (call M.D. if >200 mg/dL). Urine glucose BID • For discontinuation, PN rate to be decreased by 50% for 15 min. x2. Accucheck 30 and 60 min. after PN discontinued (central solutions only). Laboratory • Nutrition Panel I (electrolytes, BUN, creat., glu. Ca, Mg, PO_4) Day 1 & 2, then q.Mon. & Thr. • Nutrition Panel II (albumin, pre-albumin, total protein, LFTs) Day 1, then q.Monday • Triglyceride - Day 1 & 4, then q.Mon. (draw at least 4-6h after lipid infusion complete) • 24 hr urine for TUN (total urine nitrogen) on Day 4 & q.Mon

Time/Date Written: ____________ Time/Date Noted: ____________ Physician Signature: ____________ Physician (Dictation) I.D. # ____________	Addressograph

Figure 3.7.
Adult parenteral nutrition solution orders.

- Changes to the lipid emulsion order require the lipid emulsion section to be completely rewritten to limit the possibility of confusion.
- Make sure to indicate if currently infusing and previously ordered solution may be used before carrying out a new order (e.g., "begin new order with next PN solution" or "may use previously mixed solution") to avoid waste. PN orders should be delivered to or faxed to the pharmacy as soon as pos-

sible to facilitate timely implementation. There is no such thing as an emergent requirement for TPN initiation.

Standard and Custom Solutions

Standard amino acid/electrolyte solutions have been developed to meet most patients' needs. These solutions will typically provide 1.0–1.5 g/kg/day of amino acids as well as maintenance quantities of electrolytes, minerals (except iron), and vitamins when administered in sufficient volume to meet the patient's maintenance fluid requirement. Caloric and protein intake can be adjusted by adjusting the PN infusion rate. Using standard solutions is cost effective and leads to fewer errors inherent in custom making each new solution. When a designated electrolyte, mineral, or trace element concentration is greater than the standard, additional is added to the standard solution. However, when a lesser quantity of an ingredient is ordered, the solution must be prepared from "scratch." PN solutions containing specialized amino acid formulas such as the branched-chain amino acid formulas may be substantially more expensive not only for the ingredient, but because the PN solution containing these ingredients must be made custom.

To avoid confusion when nonstandard solutions are necessary, write out the quantity for all electrolytes, minerals, vitamins, and trace elements so there is no confusion as to which concentrations are standard and which are not.

Initiating Parenteral Nutrition

Peripheral Parenteral Nutrition

A 60-kg patient (IBW 55 kg) is admitted with a partial small bowel obstruction. Indication: The patient is losing 1200 ml/day via NG suction and is NPO. Indication: expect NPO > 7 days due to small bowel obstruction.

Fluid Requirements

Maintenance: 1500 + 20 ml/kg > 20 kg	2200 ml
Replacement of NG losses:	1200 ml
TOTAL	3400 ml

Protein Requirements

1–1.2 g/kg/day = 55–66 g/day

Caloric Requirements (Estimated)

33 kcal/kg/day (maintenance) (or preferably use direct calorimetry) = 1815 kcal

Suggested Regimen

1. 10% dextrose with 3.5% amino acid and standard electrolytes, minerals, vitamins, and trace elements at 100 ml/hr (2.4 l/day). This will provide 816 kcal and 84 g amino acids. Begin infusion at 100 ml/hr.
2. 20% lipid emulsion (500 ml) infused over 10 hours (50 ml/hr) with the parenteral nutrition solution to provide 1000 kcal/day. Serum triglyc-

eride concentration should be checked 4–6 hours after the lipid infusion is completed to ascertain adequate clearance.

3. The appropriate replacement solution in this setting is 5% dextrose with 0.45% saline containing 20 mEq/L KCl infused at a rate of ml/ml of NGT output (replaced every 8 hours).
4. Totals for proposed regimen:
   Calories: 1816 non-protein kcal (33 kcal/kg IBW)
   Amino acids: 84 g (1.5 g/kg IBW)
   (See Sample Parenteral Nutrition Order Form, Fig. 3.7)

Note: In small patients, peripheral parenteral nutrition can provide complete nutritional requirements.

5. Maximize chloride and minimize acetate if patient is alkalotic.

Central Parenteral Nutrition

Example: A 55-kg patient (IBW 65 kg) is admitted with severe graft versus host disease with diarrhea and protein-losing enteropathy following a bone marrow transplant. A central line (Hickman catheter) is in place. Stool output is 8 liters daily.

Indication

GVHD and diarrhea

Fluid Requirements

Maintenance: 1500 ml + 20 mL/kg IBW	= 2400 mL
Replacement of diarrheal losses	= <u>8000 mL</u>
	TOTAL 10400 mL

Protein Requirements

1.5 g/kg/day = 98 g/day
Collect stool and urine for total nitrogen loss determination; requirement may be greater.

Caloric Requirements

Since the patient is 85% of IBW, this regimen should produce weight gain.
Rebuild tissue and weight gain: 40 kcal/kg/IBW = 2600 kcal/day

Suggested Regimen

1. 25% dextrose with 4.25% amino acids with standard electrolytes, minerals, vitamins, and trace elements (additional sodium, potassium, acetate, zinc, magnesium, and/or addition of selenium may be necessary depending on serum concentrations). Infusion at 100 ml/hr (2.4 l/day) will provide 2040 kcal and 102 g amino acids.
2. The solution should be infused at 40 ml/hr for 8 hr initially and glucose concentration (Accucheck) determined after 2 hours. If the glucose is < 200 ml/dL, the infusion rate should be increased by 25 cc/hr every 8

hours (with the glucose checked 2 hours after each rate increase) until the goal rate of 100 ml/hr is obtained.

3. 20% lipid emulsion (200 ml) infused over 6 hours to provide 400 kcal/day "piggybacked" with the TPN solution. The serum triglyceride concentration should be checked 4–6 hours after the lipid infusion is completed to ascertain adequate clearance. This is especially important in this case because cyclosporin may impair triglyceride clearance.
4. Maximize acetate and minimize chloride if patient is acidotic from diarrhea.
5. The appropriate replacement solution in this setting is 0.45% saline or normal saline containing 20 mEq/L KCl infused at a rate ml/ml of diarrheal losses every 8 hours.

Totals for Proposed Regimen
Calories = 2440 non-protein kcal (39 kcal/kg IBW)
Amino Acids = 102 g (1.6 g/kg IBW)
Fluid = 10,400 ml
(See Parenteral Nutrition Order Forms, Figs. 3.7 and 3.8)

MONITORING OF PARENTERAL NUTRITION

Proper monitoring of patients receiving parenteral nutrition is essential to:

1. Detect and prevent complications.
2. Determine if proper and adequate nutritional ingredients are being infused.
3. Document positive clinical benefits.

The recommended laboratory tests and monitoring frequency are listed on the Parenteral Nutrition Order Form (Figs. 3.7, 3.8). These include:

1. Initial measured weight and height; daily weights thereafter.
2. Temperature every 8 hours.
3. Strict input and output recording.
4. Blood glucose 2 hours after each rate increase for central PN and every 6 hours until patient is stable, then urine glucose each nursing shift thereafter.
5. Baseline blood tests (before PN):
   - Electrolytes, including magnesium, calcium, phosphate
   - Glucose
   - CBC with differential and quantitative platelets
   - Fe and TIBC and/or ferritin
   - PT
   - Total serum protein, albumin, prealbumin, BUN and creatinine
   - AST, ALT, bilirubin and alkaline phosphatase
   - Triglycerides
   - Zinc, chromium, selenium or copper if clinically indicated

Adult Parenteral Nutrition Solution Orders

Baylor College of Medicine 6550 Fannin, Houston, TX 77030 **Use Ball Point Pen - Press Firmly**

Check Box:
☒ **Initiation Orders** ☐ **Change of Therapy** ☐ **Rate change only** ☐ **Discontinuation**
PN orders will not be filled by the pharmacy in the absence of indication and estimated needs unless rate change only. When change of therapy is checked, all PN solutions already made will be used unless otherwise ordered.

CONSULTS	Check Box: ☒ NST Clerk: Please notify
INDICATION FOR TPN	Graft Versus Host Disease / Diarrhea
ESTIMATED NEEDS	**Height** 5'7" inches **Current Weight** 55 kg **Ideal Body Weight** 65 kg Estimated caloric requirement 2600 kcal/day (25-35 kcal/kg/day for maintenance, 40 kcal/kg/day for repletion) Estimated protein requirement 98 g/day (1.0-1.5 g/kg/day)* *May not be appropriate in hepatic or renal failure ☐ **Check box** to order **Indirect Calorimetry** to estimate resting energy expenditure and to determine caloric requirement.

FORMULA — CHECK BOX FOR DESIRED FORMULA:

1. PERIPHERAL
☐ Dextrose 10%-Amino Acid 3.5%
(340 non-protein kcal/L) (35 g protein/L)

CENTRAL
☒ Dextrose 25%-Amino Acid 4.25%
(850 g/L non-protein kcal/L) (42.5 g protein/L)

☐ OTHER ____________

2. ELECTROLYTES Check one:

☐ **Standard Electrolytes**
Na 35 mEq/L
K 30 mEq/L Mg 10 mEq/L
Ca 5 mEq/L P 10 mMol/L

☐ **Custom Electrolytes**
(Write as totals per L)
Na ____ mEq/L
K ____ mEq/L Mg ____ mEq/L
Ca ____ mEq/L P ____ mMol/L

Chloride and Acetate
☐ Minimize Cl, max. Ac (for acidosis)
☒ Max. Cl, minimize Ac (for alkalosis)
☐ Balance CL & Ac
☐ Ac ____ Cl ____

3. VITAMINS AND TRACE ELEMENTS
Unless otherwise ordered, MVI-12, Vitamin K_1 mg/day, and Multi-trace elements (Zn 3mg, Cr 12μg, Cu 1.2mg, Se 40μg, Mn 0.3mg) will be included in each daily TPN solution. Additional supplementation should be ordered under "Other".

4. ADDITIVES
Regular Human Insulin ∅ U/L H_2 Blocker Ranitidine 150 mg/24hrs Other ____________

5. LIPID EMULSION Check Box
☐ 10% 500 ml (1.1 kcal/mL) ☒ 20% 200 ml (2.0 kcal/mL) ☐ 20% 500 ml (2.0 kcal/mL) Frequency q O

RATE	**Check one box and fill in blanks:** ☒ Start central PN at 40 mL/hr for 8 hrs, increase to 70 mL/hr for 8 hrs, then increase to 100 mL/hr thereafter (goal) ☐ Infuse at ______ mL/hr **All fat emulsion infused at 50 mL/hr**
MONITORING	Nursing • Daily weights, strict inputs and outputs, temperature every 8 hours • Accucheck 2 hrs after every rate increase, then q.6h x 3 days (call M.D. if >200 mg/dL). Urine glucose BID • For discontinuation, PN rate to be decreased by 50% for 15 min. x2. Accucheck 30 and 60 min. after PN discontinued (central solutions only). Laboratory • Nutrition Panel I (electrolytes, BUN, creat., glu. Ca, Mg, PO_4) Day 1 & 2, then q.Mon. & Thr. • Nutrition Panel II (albumin, pre-albumin, total protein, LFTs) Day 1, then q.Monday • Triglyceride - Day 1 & 4, then q.Mon. (draw at least 4-6h after lipid infusion complete) • 24 hr urine for TUN (total urine nitrogen) on Day 4 & q.Mon

Time/Date Written: 8/28/95 1100
Time/Date Noted: ____________
Physician Signature: [illegible]
Physician (Dictation) I.D. # 1234

Addressograph

Figure 3.8.
Adult parenteral nutrition solution orders (completed).

6. Tests performed daily until patient is stable (usually the first four days)
   - Electrolytes, including magnesium, calcium, phosphate
   - Glucose 2 hours after each rate increase and every 6 hours
   - BUN and creatinine

- ➢ Triglycerides—once, unless elevated, 4–6 hours after lipid infusion completed

  When the patient is stable, these blood tests should not be repeated more frequently than twice weekly, unless otherwise clinically indicated.

7. Laboratory tests performed weekly or biweekly:
   - ➢ AST, ALT, bilirubin
   - ➢ Total protein, albumin, prealbumin
   - ➢ CBC and platelets
   - ➢ Various trace elements if patient is receiving additional supplementation
   - ➢ 24 hour urine for total urine nitrogen (TUN)

Patient Cost of Parenteral Nutrition

The cost of properly monitoring parenteral nutrition and of maintaining a central venous catheter should be considered when contemplating use of parenteral nutrition therapy. Patient charges for TPN and monitoring may be more than $1,000 per day.

COMPLICATIONS OF PARENTERAL NUTRITION

Mechanical

Related to CVC Placement

Pneumothorax
Hydrothorax
Catheter embolism
Arterial puncture
Air embolism—check tubing for air
Central venous thrombosis
SVC or IVC Syndrome
Brachial plexus injury
Myocardial perforation, cardiac tamponade
Cardiac arrhythmias
Catheter malposition
Thoracic duct injury

Catheter Breakage

Silastic® long-term CVC can be repaired if damage occurs along the external segment. Such catheters should be clamped only with smooth jawed plastic occlusion forceps; saw tooth clamps will damage the catheter.

When a silastic CVC is found to be damaged, the following steps should be undertaken immediately:

1. Clamp line with preattached CVC clamps or smooth jawed occlusion forceps between the patient and the damaged segment.

2. Disinfect area of damage with alcohol and povidone iodine and wrap with a dry sterile gauze pad.
3. Attempt to instill a heparin flush as appropriate to protect patency of catheter while awaiting repair.
4. Order appropriate repair trays STAT from central supply:
   CVC specific repair kit (Hickman 1.6 mm repair kit)
   Hickman/Broviac repair tray

Catheter Occlusion

The following may indicate catheter occlusion:

1. Inability to infuse lipids even when dextrose/amino acid solution infuses
2. Difficulty flushing the CVC
3. Inability to withdraw blood from the CVC
4. Blood back flow into the IV tubing

Catheter Thrombosis

Treatment

Push administration of **urokinase** (not streptokinase) for clearing blocked central venous catheters.

Rationale

Fibrin accumulation can cause partial or complete blockage of indwelling CVCs. Administration of a small volume of urokinase, a thrombolytic agent, IV push into the CVC may clear blockage of the internal lumen of the CVC without causing a systemic change in clotting times.

Contraindications (Allergy to Urokinase)

If additional symptoms such as neck or face swelling, swelling of the limb proximal to the CVC or pain along the CVC tract with infusion exist, IV push urokinase should not be administered until a radiopaque dye study or ultrasound can be performed to rule out vascular thrombosis.

Active internal bleeding, peptic ulcer disease, recent cerebrovascular injury or intracranial/intraspinal surgery within the prior 2 months are contraindications for intravenous urokinase infusion.

Procedure

Silastic® CVCs (Hickman/Broviac-type CVCs)
Urokinase – 5,000 units/ml
– 1 ml = 5,000 units

PICC lines (with extension tubing)
0.6 ml of urokinase, 5,000 units/1 ml = 3,000 units

Subcutaneous infusion ports
2 ml of urokinase, 5,000 units/ml = 10,000 units
maximum dose is 3000 u/kg

Pediatric Catheter
1 ml of urokinase, 5000 units/ml = 5000 units

1. Reconstitute and draw up urokinase into sterile syringe (1–3 ml as appropriate); 1 ml for pediatrics.
2. Dose volume should approximate volume of inner lumen of CVC, see Appendix 1, Table 18.
3. Remove cap or IV tubing at CVC hub after cleansing hub as described under catheter care.
4. Attach urokinase syringe to CVC. Slowly instill a full dose of urokinase using a gentle push-pull motion on the plunger of the syringe into each catheter lumen. An adapter may be placed in the catheter hub.
5. Clamp CVC and leave urokinase in place for 10 minutes.
6. After 10 minutes, unclamp CVC and attempt to aspirate drug along with 3 to 5 ml of blood using a new syringe.
7. If unable to aspirate, reinstill urokinase into each lumen and clamp CVC for another 30 minutes and attempt to repeat steps 2–4 and attempt to re-aspirate in 1 hour. If still unsuccessful, repeat steps 2–4 and attempt re-aspiration in 3 hours or consult with radiology for a catheter check.
8. If successful, irrigate CVC with 3 to 5 ml of 0.9% sodium chloride, then heparin flush and cap or resume IV therapy as necessary (do not return aspirated blood).

Non-Thrombotic Occlusion

Non-thrombotic catheter occlusions may be caused by poor solubility of calcium, phosphorus, and other divalent cations. Check PN formulation with pharmacy.

- If urokinase is unsuccessful in restoring catheter patency, non-thrombotic occlusion should be considered. Hydrochloric acid (HCl) may be useful in clearing mineral precipitate (17).
- 0.2–0.5 ml of sterile 0.1 N HCl is instilled using a 1-ml syringe. Re-prep catheter up. Wait 20 minutes and attempt to aspirate. This may be repeated two more times if necessary. Leave HCl in the catheter for 1–3 hours before attempting to re-aspirate. If successful, flush the catheter with 3–5 ml of 0.9% sodium chloride followed by a heparin flush.

Infections

Central catheters become infected at three sites: skin entry site, the catheter hub, and the fibrin sheath coating the outside of the catheter inside the vein.

Catheter Sepsis

This is the greatest concern in patients receiving parenteral nutrition since an indwelling catheter is a potential conduit for organism entry from skin contamination, and a malnourished or debilitated patient may be immunocompromised and, therefore, is a good host for infection. Using aseptic and following prescribed catheter care protocols are essential for minimizing infections.

Evaluation of Fever

- If any fever greater than 38.5°C develops during the administration of parenteral nutrition, close examination for a focal source must be undertaken. Fever may also be associated with allergic reactions to the nutrients (rare), other drugs, or contaminated solutions (rare).
- Blood cultures for bacteria and fungi should be obtained both from the catheter and peripheral vein. Sterile technique is particularly important. Also check CBC with differential, urine and chest radiograph.
- Antibiotics should usually be withheld unless it is clinically obvious the patient has a catheter infection (e.g., rigors after flushing catheter), the patient continues to spike a fever for more than 8 hours, or progresses to septic shock. The PN nutrition solution should be held, but alternative electrolyte solutions should still be administered if necessary through a *new* catheter. If the patient defervesces with holding the nutrient solution and re-spikes a fever with continuation of parenteral nutrition, that suggests either the catheter or the solution is the source. Samples of the nutrient solution should be sent for culture. Remember that sepsis can occur in the absence of fever or leukocytosis. If the catheter is a temporary (non-Hickman, "Broviac") type, it should be removed and the tip sent for culture and broad spectrum aerobic gram positive and negative antibiotic coverage should be initiated. Vancomycin and an aminoglycoside or third generation cephalosporin are started as empiric coverage to cover for *Staphylococcus epidermidis, S. aureus,* and *E. coli,* the most common infecting organisms. Pseudomonas is not uncommonly an infecting organism. Patients receiving parenteral nutrition may occasionally be infected with unusual organisms, and these should not necessarily be dismissed as contaminants. Quantitative blood cultures obtained from the catheter may be useful.
- Antibiotic therapy can be tailored to an individual organism once a positive identification and sensitivity are available. Fastidious gram negative organisms may require up to 4 days for growth to be detected in culture media. Because of the potential toxicity of anti-fungal therapy, no empiric use of amphotericin is indicated unless yeast are detected on the peripheral blood smear. If catheter-associated sepsis is documented, the catheter should be removed if it is a temporary catheter and antibiotics infused for 7 days. Fungal infections require 250–500 mg of amphotericin over the total course of therapy. A new catheter can be placed and parenteral nutrition resumed once the patient has been afebrile on antibiotics at least 48 hours.
- Every attempt should be made to preserve Hickman and Broviac type

catheters. Catheter-associated sepsis can often be treated successfully by leaving the catheter *in situ* (18). That is especially important for a patient requiring permanent TPN who may have few sites for venous access. However, antibiotics must be infused for 14–28 days. If the patient remains febrile 72 hours after antibiotic therapy is initiated or develops progression of the sepsis syndrome, (including but not limited to renal, respiratory, or cardiac failure, DIC, endocarditis, or embolism), the catheter should be removed immediately. The catheter must always be removed in the event of a systemic fungal infection. For patients requiring home TPN, antibiotics can also be infused at home although only daily to twice daily regimens are feasible. The patient can be trained by the nursing staff/nutrition support nurse and home health nurses to do this.

Exit and Tunnel Site Infections

These infections usually occur in the absence of fever or leukocytosis. They are identified by local tenderness, purulent exudate and/or erythema at the catheter exit site. Temporary catheters should be removed and the exudate cultured. The usual organisms are *S. aureus* or *S. epidermidis* and intravenous vancomycin should be initiated pending culture results. Antibiotics should be continued for 5–7 days even in the absence of positive cultures. In the event of an infected Hickman or Broviac type catheter, an attempt should be made to treat the catheter *in situ* with intravenous vancomycin. One to two weeks of antibiotic therapy are usually necessary, and the success rate is approximately 50%. Care should be taken to exclude a *tunnel infection*. This is an infection of the subcutaneous tunnel that the catheter follows under the skin. This infection cannot be treated without catheter removal. It is indicated by a red streak and tenderness of the skin overlying the tunnel tract.

Metabolic Complications

Hyperglycemia

If a patient spills 2+ or greater glucose in the urine on two or more consecutive occasions or blood glucose is 200 mg/dL:

- The usual initiation rate should be approximately 2–3 mg/kg/min of dextrose (i.e., 40 ml/hr for D25).
- Consider drug interactions with the test system.
- Verify the infusion rate and ensure that no "catching up" has been attempted in the event the patient may have missed a portion of his daily parenteral nutrition.
- Check serum potassium. Glucosuria may be secondary to hypokalemia, and this can be corrected without insulin administration.
- Check for sepsis or other infections. Hyperglycemia may often occur prior to fever. Chromium deficiency has been poorly documented in humans and has been only possibly described in three case reports. Therefore, it is extremely unlikely that chromium deficiency would account for the hyperglycemia.
- Should it be necessary to add insulin, initially add 1 unit per 10 g dextrose

(e.g., 10 units for D10W). Orders should be written to cover the patient with a sliding scale insulin dosing in the event that 1 unit per 10 g dextrose is insufficient. Additional insulin can be added to the next TPN bottle. It is inappropriate to regulate the patient's serum glucose below 150 mg/dL unless symptomatic from glucosuria. Finer control is rarely possible and places the patient at risk for hypoglycemia. If hyperglycemia persists despite the use of > 2.0 units insulin per g dextrose, the level of dextrose infusion should be decreased. An attempt should be made to gradually decrease the insulin dose once blood glucose concentrations are consistently ≤ 120 mg/dL.

- The daily urine volume can be multiplied by the energy value of glucose (3.75 kcal/g) to estimate the energy loss from glucosuria.

Hypoglycemia

- Hypoglycemia may occur with abrupt cessation of central PN. Therefore, concentrated dextrose infusions (> 10%) should be tapered before cessation.
- Tapering may be performed by decreasing the PN rate by 50% for 15 minutes, and then another 50% for 15 minutes, then disconnect. For the rare patients who develop hypoglycemia after this tapering, future taperings can be extended to 45 to 60 minutes. It is for this reason the blood glucose should be checked 30 and 60 minutes after TPN with a < 10% dextrose concentration is discontinued.
- In a "Code Blue" situation, PN should be immediately discontinued and 10% dextrose simultaneously substituted.
- Hypoglycemia may occasionally be the initial manifestation of sepsis even in the absence of fever or leukocytosis.

Electrolyte Imbalances

The most common electrolyte imbalances are related to potassium, phosphorus, and magnesium. Abnormalities in serum calcium occur less commonly. During protein synthesis, the serum concentration of these ions may decrease (see re-feeding syndrome).

- Hyperchloremic metabolic acidosis may be treated by the substitution of acetate for the chloride salts of sodium and potassium. The underlying cause of metabolic acidosis or alkalosis should be corrected before manipulating the parenteral nutrition solution. Bicarbonate itself may not be added to parenteral nutrition solutions due to incompatibilities. Abnormalities in serum calcium occur less commonly.
- The tendency to "chase" slight variations in lab tests with frequent changes in the electrolyte content of parenteral nutrition solutions is to be avoided because this is expensive and leads to waste. Whenever possible, deficiencies should be corrected with separate "piggybacked" bolus infusions. Stable, increased electrolyte requirements may be met by addition to the parenteral nutrition solution. Sources of electrolyte loss such as nasogastric suction, diarrhea or fistula drainage should be identified and replaced separately from

PN. Most important, iatrogenic electrolyte abnormalities can be minimized by appropriate monitoring, especially when the PN solution is changed.

Elevated BUN

Elevated BUN may be caused by either catabolism due to insufficient calories and/or protein, or excessive protein intake. The differential diagnosis should also include dehydration, renal insufficiency, and gastrointestinal hemorrhage. Drug therapy should be re-evaluated in situations where an elevated BUN is encountered.

Hepatic Aminotransferase Elevation

Elevation of ALT, AST, and/or alkaline phosphatase may occur 2–14 days after initiating parenteral nutrition. The ALT and AST return to normal or near normal without discontinuing the parenteral nutrition. Alkaline phosphatase may remain mildly elevated due to the cholestatic effects of parenteral nutrition, biliary sludge (which occurs in 100% of patients receiving parenteral nutrition in the complete absence of oral intake after 4 weeks), a calculous cholecystitis, or cholecystitis or metabolic bone disease. A normal or low alkaline phosphatase may be associated with zinc deficiency.

Elevation of ALT and/or AST may be related to overfeeding, excessive dextrose infusion, excessive lipid infusion, choline deficiency, medications or preexisting liver disease such as chronic hepatitis. The bilirubin is seldom elevated in adults. Over the short-term, liver test abnormalities are usually without consequence although right upper quadrant pain secondary to hepatic steatosis may occur. Chronic liver disease secondary to parenteral nutrition, while common in neonates, is uncommon in adults until the patient has received several years of parenteral nutrition.

Cholecystitis

Cholecystitis or acalculous cholecystitis may occur in up to 40% of patients receiving long-term parenteral nutrition. Most gallstones are cholesterol stones, and there is a relationship with decreased gallbladder motility and decreased CCK release; 100% of patients receiving TPN will have biliary sludge after 4 weeks. It is therefore important to encourage some oral intake if at all possible. The use of parenteral CCK is expensive and occasionally associated with nausea, vomiting, and abdominal pain.

Delayed Gastric Emptying

Both dextrose/amino acid solutions and lipid emulsions have been associated with delayed gastric emptying and perhaps early satiety. This effect may persist for some period even after TPN is discontinued.

Lipoprotein Abnormalities

An elevation in serum triglycerides may be seen because of the lipid infusion. Serum concentrations $>$ 250 mg/dL may lead to impairment of the reticular endothelial system. Impaired triglyceride clearance may occur in renal failure or with the use of cyclosporin; it does not occur during cirrhosis. Serum triglycerides ≥ 1000 mg/dL may cause pancreatitis and, therefore should definitely be avoided. The rate and total infusion of lipid emulsion should be reduced as necessary although a minimum of 2–4% of total calories as linoleic acid must be provided to prevent essential fatty acid deficiency. Serum triglycerides should be measured 4–6 hours after lipid infusion has been completed. If an elevated concentration is found, the phlebotomy time should be determined to ascertain if it occurred during the lipid infusion. In contrast to triglycerides, hypocholesterolemia often occurs during TPN, although both LDL and HDL are equally affected. No known abnormalities related to this have been described although the effects on wound healing are unknown.

Metabolic Bone Disease

Osteopenia is a characteristic of patients receiving long-term parenteral nutrition. It is a heterogenous disease and may include either osteoporosis or osteomalacia and may be associated with bone pain. A correlation with serum fluoride concentration has been identified in humans but fluoride supplementation is currently not approved or recommended. Aluminum contamination of parenteral nutrition solutions was a problem before 1986. Some patients receiving parenteral nutrition may have elevated parathyroid hormone (PTH) with resultant osteoporosis, probably because of insufficient calcium infusion or renal insufficiency although others have normal or suppressed PTH. The etiology of metabolic bone disease during parenteral nutrition is the subject of ongoing investigation.

Renal Insufficiency

Decreased glomerular filtrate rate has been observed in patients receiving long-term parenteral nutrition. The etiology may be partly related to excessive chromium infusion and systemic infections, but is mostly undefined (19).

Refeeding Syndrome

If nutritional repletion is over-vigorous or achieved too rapidly in severely malnourished patients, refeeding syndrome may result. The serum phosphate concentration may decrease dramatically because of the intracellular movement of the ion for ATP production. The result can be hemolysis, cardiac dysfunction, neuromuscular dysfunction including sensory loss, paralysis, seizures, rhabdomyolysis, and respiratory failure (20). Serum potassium and magnesium may also decrease abruptly because of intracellular shifts. Therefore, nutritional repletion, especially with carbohydrate energy sources, should proceed gingerly over the first week with serum phosphate, potassium and magnesium determined daily. There may be additional safety value in using a high protein formula for repletion at this time.

Initiating nutritional therapy too rapidly may also lead to fluid overload, increased metabolic rate, and subsequent congestive heart failure. The body adapts to starvation by lowering resting energy expenditure. If the patient is well below IBW, use *actual* body weight to calculate initial nutritional requirements and set reasonable caloric goals (i.e., 30–35 kcal/kg/day). It may be wise to begin parenteral as well as enteral nutrition therapy with as little as 20 kcal/kg/day IBW in a severely malnourished patient. Indirect calorimetry should be performed if possible on all severely malnourished patients because estimates of caloric requirements in this setting may have a significant degree of inaccuracy, and miscalculation can lead to undesirable patient outcome in this group. It is prudent to initially restrict dextrose calories to reflect endogenous glucose synthetic rate (2 mg/kg/min or 150–200 g/day) to avoid hyperglycemia and hyperinsulinemia, the latter of which will lead to further decreases in serum potassium concentration. The increased serum insulin also promotes an antidiuretic effect, which can lead to fluid overload and further cardiac decompensation. The level of protein repletion does not need to be decreased.

Overfeeding

The provision of more than 40 kcal/kg IBW/day will not accelerate protein and tissue synthesis. Overfeeding can cause significant metabolic complications including hepatic steatosis, hyperglycemia, and excessive CO_2 production. The latter may precipitate respiratory failure or inhibit successful ventilator weaning in patients with marginal respiratory reserve. Severe and potentially life-threatening hypophosphatemia, hypokalemia, and/or hypomagnesemia may also develop.

Intestinal Morphology and Functional Changes

Frank intestinal atrophy associated with the use of TPN and lack of oral or enteral intake has not been demonstrated in humans. TPN is associated with a decrease in villus height and an increase in intestinal permeability in man. However, the clinical significance of this finding is currently undefined in humans.

HOME TPN

Assessment and Training

- Requires proper training of the patient or significant other in proper catheter care techniques, use of an IV pump, preparation of TPN solutions for infusion, and IV antibiotic use (if necessary). Do not discharge the patient home until they have demonstrated safety and proficiency in their personal care.
- Family members can often be trained to prepare the solutions and to connect and disconnect the TPN. Alternatively, a social worker may be successful in finding a suitable trainee but is often unsuccessful, and this will involve additional, often unreimbursed expenditures.
- The capability of the patient for family for home TPN should be properly assessed before referral. This includes:

  - Patient or significant other manual dexterity, aptitude and compliance
  - Home environment including location, site of solution preparation, overall cleanliness, designated extra refrigerator
  - Indication for home TPN including progression or prognosis of the underlying disease
- Requires the patient to be metabolically stable without requiring frequent adjustment in their TPN prior to hospital discharge.
- Early referral of potential home TPN patients allows for a smoother transition. For example, patients with endstage cancer who are bedridden expected to live only 1–2 months may not be appropriate candidates.
- Family or significant other support.
- Finances. Home TPN can be extraordinarily expensive (well over $100,000 per year). Alternative financial sources may require early exploration.

Preparation for Discharge

- The hours of TPN infusion should be "cycled" or compressed into a nighttime infusion schedule prior to discharge (see cycling TPN order form, Fig. 3.9). This permits the patient to perform usual activity during the day (including gainful employment!) and to receive TPN overnight while asleep. See TPN cycling schedule (Table 3.3).
- A 10–12 hour infusion cycle is usually the goal. The infusion period is compressed while the total infusion volume remains unchanged. Some patients may require a slower infusion rate and longer infusion time because of the inability to tolerate the fluid load.
- The blood glucose (Accucheck is acceptable) should be checked 2 hours into each infusion period that the rate is increased. The addition of regular insulin to the PN solution is sometimes necessary. Insulin should not be added to the PN solution once it is already infusing.
- To taper TPN, reduce the rate by 50% for 15 minutes, and then by another 50% for another 15 minutes before it is discontinued. The taper period may be extended to 45 to 60 minutes with smaller incremental rate reductions for patients who develop hypoglycemia with the standard taper.
- Tapering is not included in the infusion time.
- Blood glucose should also be checked 30 and 60 minutes after the PN is tapered off because the high concentration dextrose infusion (at rapid rate especially) stimulates insulin secretion and may result in "reactive" hypoglycemia. The body "adapts" to this phenomenon on a more chronic basis, and once the blood glucose is acceptable after the tapering, home monitoring is seldom necessary unless the patient develops symptoms of hypoglycemia. It may also be necessary to decrease the dextrose concentration if the blood glucose cannot be satisfactorily controlled. Patients can be taught to add insulin to the TPN solution, but this should only be done when preparing the solution only (prior to hanging the bag).
- The PN solution at home consists of a single 2–3 liter bag, which may differ from that used in the hospital. Three-in-one bags, in which the lipid emulsion is combined with the dextrose/amino acid formula are becoming

TPN Cycling Orders

Baylor College of Medicine 6550 Fannin, Houston, TX 77030 **Use Ball Point Pen - Press Firmly**

CYCLING: The process of changing the TPN regimen from a continuous infusion to a shortened, fixed infusion. It is generally suggested to compress the total 24h volume of TPN by 2h increments for each subsequent 24h period.

WEANING OFF TPN: Decrease infusion rate by half for 15 minutes; again decrease infusion rate by half for 15 minutes; stop TPN, flush and cap lumen. Fat infusion to run over same time duration as TPN.

Cycling orders as follows:

Present TPN is infused @_________ ml/Hr over 24 hours QD providing ____________ ml/day

DAY 1: Beginning ____________ (Date), ____________ (Day) start compression
Discontinue TPN ____________ (Time)
RESTART TPN @ ___________ (Time), @ _____________ (Rate) ml/h

DAY 2: On _____________ (Date), COMPRESS TPN @ ____________ (Time)
RESTART TPN @ ___________ (Time), @ _____________ (Rate) ml/h

DAY 3: On _____________ (Date), COMPRESS TPN @ ____________ (Time)
RESTART TPN @ ___________ (Time), @ _____________ (Rate) ml/h

DAY 4: On _____________ (Date), COMPRESS TPN @ ____________ (Time)
RESTART TPN @ ___________ (Time), @ _____________ (Rate) ml/h

DAY 5: On _____________ (Date), COMPRESS TPN @ ____________ (Time)
RESTART TPN @ ___________ (Time), @ _____________ (Rate) ml/h

DAY 6: On _____________ (Date), COMPRESS TPN @ ____________ (Time)
RESTART TPN @ ___________ (Time), @ _____________ (Rate) ml/h

DAY 7: On _____________ (Date), COMPRESS TPN @ ____________ (Time)
RESTART TPN @ ___________ (Time), @ _____________ (Rate) ml/h

- After desired rate is achieved, continue cycling schedule as ordered on day _______.

Once each day, after stopping the TPN, flush each lumen of the central line with HEPARIN 100 units. Chart time and number of lumens on the MAR.

OBTAIN ACCUCHECK _____ hours and _____ hours after restarting TPN for _____ days. Also obtain accuchecks 30 min. and one hour after the end of infusion.

OTHER INSTRUCTIONS

Time/Date Written: ____________ Time/Date Noted: ____________ Physician Signature: ____________ Physician (Dictation) I.D. #:	**Addressograph:**

Figure 3.9.
TPN cycling orders.

Table 3.3.
TPN Compression Schedule

Day	1l/night Rate	1l/night Hours	2l/night Rate	2l/night Hours	3l/night Rate	3l/night Hours
1	42 ml/hr	24	83 ml/hr	24	125 ml/hr	24
2	45	22	90	22	136	22
3	50	20	100	20	150	20
4	55	18	111	18	166	18
5	62	16	125	16	187	16
6	71	14	142	14	214	14
7	83	12	166	12	250	12
8	100	10	200	10	300	10

increasingly popular. However, the patient or significant other must carefully inspect the bag for cracking or creaming of the emulsion prior to use. Alternatively, the lipid emulsion may be "piggybacked" into the TPN line.

- The solution comes premixed from the pharmacy. However, the patient or significant other must add the vitamin preparation immediately before use because some vitamins may destabilize especially if exposed to light over time. The patient or significant other can be taught to add other additives including H2 blockers or insulin if necessary. The number of additives that the patient is required to add in the home environment should be minimized. It is wise to use as few additives as possible. Each additional entry into the bag creates additional work and inconvience, and worse, may increase the risk of poor technique and increase the risk of infection.
- Daily TPN and/or infusion may not be required for some patients who may have sufficient absorption to allow for partial TPN support (3–6 times weekly for instance).

Complications

- There is a significant risk of biliary sludge formation and the development of gallstones associated with long-term TPN. Therefore, patients should be allowed and encouraged to eat some if possible, even if their absorption is negligible. Most patients will prefer to eat simply for the pleasure involved, but oral food intake will help to stimulate gallbladder contractivity and prevent sludge formation. Some oral intake may also be advisable to prevent intestinal complications associated with TPN although the clinical significance of this is yet unclear.
- Patients or significant others should be instructed that the first sign of catheter occlusion may be the inability to infuse the lipid emulsion. They should contact their physician if difficulty with the TPN infusion is encountered.
- Patients or significant others should be instructed that the first manifestation of sepsis may occur when chills are encountered while hooking up or

flushing the catheter after disconnection. They should immediately contact their physician. Patients should also check the catheter site daily for redness or purulent drainage.

- If fever develops during the TPN infusion, the patient or significant other should be instructed to taper the TPN off in the usual manner, contact the physician who should be familiar with infections associated with central venous catheters and the treatment, and report immediately to the emergency room or clinic.
- Patients may occasionally experience muscle cramping during the TPN infusion. This may be due to intra- and extravascular electrolyte shifts and is usually alleviated by decreasing the infusion rate. This will require a longer infusion period.
- Dehydration can occur with TPN if hyperglycemia develops or appropriate additional replacement fluids are not infused. Patients with short gut syndrome, chronic diarrhea, or high output fistulas, for instance, may require additional replacement fluid, which can usually be infused simultaneously with the TPN—either as part of the TPN bag or separately in a "piggybacked" manner. This requires additional patient or significant other instruction.

References

1. Makarewicz PA, Freeman JB, Fairfull-Smith R. Prevention of superficial phlebitis during peripheral parenteral nutrition. Am J Surg 1986;151:126.
2. Tishe MS, Wong C, Martin IG, et al. Do heparin, hydrocortisone, and glyceryl trinitrate influence thrombophlebitis during full intravenous nutrition via a peripheral vein? JPEN 1995;19:507–509.
3. Cano N, Labastie-Coeyrehourq J, Lacombe P, et al. Perdialytic parenteral nutrition with lipids and amino acids in malnourished hemodialysis patients. Am J Clin Nutr 1990;52:726–730.
4. Piraino AJ, Firpo JJ, Powers DV. Prolonged hyperalimentation in catabolic chronic dialysis therapy patients. [Review]. JPEN 1981;5:463–477.
5. Pesola GR, Hogg JE, Eissa N, et al. Hypertonic nasogastric tube feedings: do they cause diarrhea? Crit Care Med 1990;18:1073–1079.
6. N Engl J Med 1992;327:1062–1068.
7. JPEN 1989;13:545–553.
8. Am J Surg 1986;151:126.
9. Crit Care Med 1990;18:327–335.
10. Crit Care Med 1979;7:113–116.
11. Crit Care Med 1980;8:73–80.
12. Ford EG, Jennings LM, Andrassy RS. Serum albumin pressure correlates with enteral feeding tolerance in the pediatric surgical patient. J Ped Surg 1987;22:597–599.
13. Zagoren AJ, Weters DW, Beck S, et al. Colloid osmoic pressure: sensitive predictor of enteral feeding tolerance. JACN 1984;3:260.
14. Patterson ML, Dominguez JM, Lyman B, et al. Enteral feeding in the hypoalbuminemic patient. JPEN 1990;14:362–365.

15. Foley EF, Borlase BC, Dzik WH, et al. Albumin-supplementation in the critically ill: A prospective, randomized trial. Arch Surg 1990;125:739–742.
16. Surg Gynecol Obstet 1986;163:359–362.
17. J Peds 1989;114:1002.
18. Buchman Al, Moukarzel A, Goodson B, et al. Catheter-related infections associated with home parenteral nutrition and predictive factors for the need for catheter removal in their treatment. JPEN 1994;18:297–302.
19. Kim Eh, Cohen RS, Ramachandran P, et al. Adhesion of percutaneously inserted Silastic central venous lines to the vein wall associated with Malassezia furfur infection. JPEN 1993;17:458–460.
20. Solomon SM, Kirby DF. The refeeding syndrome: a review. JPEN 1990;14:90–97.

CHAPTER 4

Enteral Nutrition

TRANSITION TO ENTERAL NUTRITION

Long-term disuse of the gastrointestinal tract leads to a decrease in villus height after 2 weeks and may lead to intestinal atrophy over long periods. Therefore, when TPN has been used exclusively for more than 2 weeks, the return to oral or enteral (tube feeding) nutrition should be gradual. Parenteral nutrition should be continued until the patient can be 50–75% supported with oral or enteral feeding but should be tapered to allow for the hypocaloric stimulation of appetite. The amount of lipid emulsion should be reduced first because it has more effect on appetite suppression and gastric emptying than thalamic controls or dextrose and amino acids.

Tube feeding, when using small bore (8–10 F) nasogastric feeding tubes, may serve as transitional feeding when parenteral support is being tapered. Enteral nutrition support is preferable to the parenteral route when possible because it is safer, more economical, more nutritionally complete and maintains gut structure and integrity.

INDICATIONS AND CONTRAINDICATIONS

The old dictum, "if the gut works, use it," still applies. All patients with functioning gastrointestinal tracts who are unable to orally ingest adequate nutrients to meet their nutritional requirements can benefit from supplemental or tube feeding.

Indications include:

1. Protein calorie malnutrition (inadequate oral intake of nutrients for the 5 days prior or normal nutrition status but with inadequate oral intake for the previous 7–10 days)
2. CNS disorders: comatose state, CVA, Parkinson's disease
3. Neoplasms, especially at least a 2-month prognosis, head and neck carcinoma: nutritional supplementation becomes an ethical concern.
4. Gastrointestinal disease: Crohn's disease, gastroparesis (jejunal feedings), malabsorption, short bowel syndrome (<100 cm jejunum remaining), chronic pancreatitis, possibly severe acute pancreatitis (jejunal feedings), pseudo-obstruction, scleroderma, low output distal enterocutaneous fistulas.
5. Psychiatric disorders: Severe depression, anorexia nervosa.

Contraindications to enteral feeding include:

1. Adynamic ileus
2. Complete intestinal or colonic obstruction
3 Intractable vomiting
4. Proximal high output enterocutaneous fistulas, active gastrointestinal bleeding, and shock. Diarrhea with or without malabsorption may be a contraindication and may possibly be manageable by an adjustment in enteral nutrition flow rate or formula selection.

FEEDING TUBES

Nasoenteric Feeding Tube

Preferably a small bore, 8–10 Fr feeding tube should be used. Larger tubes such as the Salem® sump have significant rates of esophageal reflux, ulcer, and stricture formation associated with long-term use, to say nothing of patient discomfort (1). Risks associated with even small bore tube placement include pneumomediastinum, bronchopleural fistula, pneumothorax, and hydrothorax. There is no evidence that fine bore feeding tubes precipitate variceal bleeding in patients with cirrhosis.

Placement should be either in the stomach or the duodenum (or lower). The risk of aspiration is not necessarily decreased with duodenal feeding (2). However, if duodenal feeding is desired, there is no efficacy in the adjunctive use of metoclopramide, except in the patient with diabetes (3). However, preliminary studies using erythromycin have suggested the potential benefit of this medication in assuring duodenal placement.

Verify proper tube placement of the tube *radiologically* before initiating feeding. Physical examination, including auscultatory confirmation, is inaccurate for determining correct tube placement (4).

Percutaneously Placed (PEG) or Surgically Placed Gastrostomy Tube

For long-term enteral feeding, gastrostomy tube placement offers no advantages over nasoenteric feeding with respect to patient nutrition, performance, or survival (5). It eliminates the replacement of the nasoenteric tube every 6 weeks. A PEG is less easily dislodged and is more comfortable for the patient. The incidence of nasoesophageal erosion and sinusitis decreases as compared with a nasoenteric feeding tube. There is no decrease in the aspiration risk. Complications do include stomal leakage, tube migration, gastric perforation, bleeding, and wound infection, the latter occurring in $< 4\%$ of patients.

Jejunostomy tubes require surgical placement, as jejunostomy tubes placed through a PEG invariably flip back into the duodenum or stomach. There are reports of direct percutaneous jejunostomy tube placement, but such a procedure is not accepted at the present time and certainly invites the risk of bowel perforation during the procedure.

Needle-Catheter Jejunostomy

A needle-catheter jejunostomy (NCJ) is easily placed during most abdominal or chest operations and may permit the early introduction of enteral feeding in the hospitalized patient. Catheter dislodgement with intraperitoneal formula leakage occurs in $< 2\%$ of patients and can be prevented simply by suturing the catheter to the abdominal wall (6, 7). The NCJ is not associated with volvulus or intestinal obstruction (8). Standard jejunostomy tubes for long-term feeding may also be surgically placed. Endoscopically placed jejunostomy tubes usually migrate back into the stomach or occlude partially because of their small lumens; they are not recommended.

FORMULA SELECTION

Considerations

a. *Patient diagnosis, nutritional status, and related concerns such as the presence of congestive heart failure, renal or hepatic insufficiency, or hypermetabolic state.*
b. *Purpose of the formula*. Oral supplementation where palatability is a concern versus tube feeding where taste is not an issue. Formulas consisting of intact proteins are more palatable (see Enteral Nutrition form).
c. *Patient's Digestive and Absorptive Ability.* Patients with acute pancreatitis may require feeding with a very low fat containing formula (Vivonex TEN®). Patients with Crohn's disease or malabsorption states may warrant a trial of enteral feeding using a readily available form of protein (free amino acids or short chain peptides) rather than intact protein found in standard formulas. These formulas are substantially more expensive than standard formulas. There is evidence, however, that the use of elemental formulas may not be superior to polymeric formulas in Crohn's disease. Chemically defined formulas are substantially more expensive than standard formulas.
d. *Formula Osmolality*. The osmolality of a formula may have a direct effect on gastrointestinal side effects and thereby tolerance to enteral therapy. Hyperosmolar formulas have an osmolality of . 300 mOsm/kg water. A starter regimen consisting of a diluted formula may be used initially in patients who have had limited oral or enteral nutrient intake in the prior 5–7 days. Once the goal rate is achieved, the formula concentration can be increased to full strength. Otherwise, intragastric hyperosmolar formula may precipitate feeding intolerance. Some studies have shown that "starter regimens" are unnecessary (9, 10). Although,

these results may only apply to patients who have had significant recent enteral or oral intake. Jejunal feeding tolerance, on the other hand, is related to the rate of infusion rather than osmolality.

e. *Cost.* Specialty formulas cost considerably more than standard isotonic formulas.

Categories of Formulas

Nutritionally Complete Formulas

These formulas are composed of protein, carbohydrate, and fat in high molecular weight form and, therefore, have lower osmolality. These formulas require normal digestive and lipolytic activity and are also less expensive. Most of these formulas are lactose free and provide 1 kcal/ml. Formulas with higher caloric density (1.5–2.0 kcal/ml) are available for use in patients who are fluid restricted. Lower sodium and potassium containing formulas and higher protein containing formulas are also available. Isotonic formulas should <u>never</u> be diluted.

Chemically Defined Formulas

These formulas have a low residue and use free amino acids or peptides as a protein source. Oligosaccharides or monosaccharides provide the carbohydrate source and most contain medium as well as long chain triglycerides. These formulas are hyperosmolar, although some are only minimally hyperosmolar and can be infused into the stomach undiluted. Dilution is unnecessary for jejunal feeding. Chemically defined formulas do not require proteolytic capacity, and Vivonex TEN® does not require lipolytic activity. Because of the low fat content of Vivonex TEN®, exclusive use can lead to essential fatty acid deficiency over an extended period. Theoretically, intestinal absorption of formulas containing di- and tripeptides may be facilitated over those containing crystalline amino acids, although this has not been conclusively demonstrated. In addition, improved absorption does not mean that increased nitrogen will be available for protein synthesis or to improve nitrogen balance (11). All chemically defined formulas are expensive and should be limited to use in research applications and in patients with malabsorption (fat malabsorption, refractory sprue, extremely short bowel syndrome), pancreatitis, or Crohn's disease (12, 13). Routine use, even in the hypoalbuminemic patient, is unwarranted. (14–16). Routine use of <u>intact</u> protein formulas may actually lead to a lower incidence of diarrhea in postoperative patients who have undergone upper gastrointestinal tract surgery (17).

Modular Formulas

These formulas are not nutritionally complete because they contain single nutrients such as carbohydrate, fat, or protein. They can be added to standard enteral products but are usually unnecessary and create additional work for Food and Nutrition Services when various complete products are available. Modular formulas include ProMod® protein powder (0.2g/ml dry volume or 3 g/tbsp), liquid carbohydrate (0.63 or 2.5 kcal/ml), corn oil (1 g fat containing 0.6 g linoleic acid with 5.4 kcal/ml) and MCT oil (7.7 kcal/ml).

Specialty Formulas

Specialty formulas are available for use in patients with a variety of clinical conditions including renal, respiratory, hepatic insufficiency, diabetes, hypermetabolic states, immunocompromised states, and fat or carbohydrate absorption. There is limited literature describing the use of many of these products. There is even less data supporting the efficacy of many of these formulas. There is limited to no efficacy information available for many of these relatively expensive formulas (15, 18, 19). Therefore, careful consideration should be given when contemplating the use of any of these formulas outside of a research setting.

There is also little efficacy for the use of fiber-containing formula even to prevent diarrhea in the critically ill (20), although this may be related to the use of soy polysaccharide instead of pectin in the formulas. Additional research may yet demonstrate the utility of using fiber-containing formulas in selected patient groups. Soy fiber may improve glucose tolerance.

There is some clinical efficacy in the use of Hepatic-Aid®. There is some clinical efficacy in the use of a hepatic failure formula (a high-branched chain, low aromatic amino acid containing formula) in chronic hepatic encephalapathy. Patients who would otherwise be unable to ingest a sufficient level of protein without precipitating a worsening of the encephalopathy may benefit from supplementation with this product (21).

Rate of Administration

Continuous

The volume and rate of formula infusion should be individually determined for each patient based on estimated caloric requirements by equations or indirect calorimetry and estimated protein requirements, confirmed with nitrogen balance studies. Isotonic formulas never require dilution. Unless there has been recent prior feeding, continuous drip infusion is preferred over intermittent feedings because initially, a rapid rate of feeding (especially for jejunal feeding) may produce cramping and diarrhea. If there is any question about the patient's digestive and/or absorptive capacity, 24-hour continuous infusion is preferred. To avoid uncontrolled changes in flow rate, an enteral feeding pump is recommended.

Tube feedings into the stomach should be initiated at isotonic strength at a rate of 40 ml/hr. If the patient tolerates this regimen, the rate can then be increased by 25 ml/hr every 8–12 hours as tolerated until the prescribed goal is met. Jejunal feeding may require initial rates as low as 10 ml/hr, especially in the immediate postoperative patient. In this situation, gastroparesis may otherwise completely preclude the use of nasogastric feeding. If nausea, vomiting, cramping, or diarrhea occur, the rate of administration should be decreased or, in gastric feedings, the concentration can be decreased. Avoid altering both rate and concentration simultaneously.

Intermittent Feedings

Intermittent feedings can be used if there has been no history of diarrhea or malabsorption, and the gastrointestinal tract is intact.

Bolus Feeding

Bolus infusions can be administered 3–5 times daily. They do not require a pump and simulate normal food intake more effectively than continuous feeding, at least in terms of gallbladder motility. Bolus feeding is most useful with a gastrostomy tube and should never be used in jejunal feeding. The formula should be administered at a drip rate or via syringe injection not exceeding 240 ml/30 minutes. Use a 100-ml bolus initially and increase the volume by 50 ml daily as tolerated. Orders should be written to specify the number of feedings and the volume to be administered over a specified period. Diarrhea is more common with bolus feeding than with continuous feeding, so consideration must be given to the individual's gastric storage and emptying capacity before considering bolus feeding (22).

Cyclic, Intermittent Feeding

Like TPN, continuous drip feeding can be compressed or "cycled" into a 10–12 overnight feeding. Night time feeding may also be used at home for supplemental feeding in patients with active Crohn's disease or other malabsorption conditions. The patient or significant other is trained to intubate their stomach with a nasoenteric tube nightly. In most cases, this is not recommended because of the possibility of improper tube placement. Night time feeding may also be used with gastrostomy but *not* with jejunostomy tube feeding.

Fluid Requirements

No formula provides sufficient free water to meet a patient's daily fluid requirement. The recommended daily water requirement in the absence of hepatic, renal, or cardiac disease is 1 ml/kcal. Most 1 kcal/ml formulas contain approximately 75% water. Therefore, patients without fluid restriction should receive enough additional free water to equal at least 25% of the total formula volume (i.e., for 2000 ml of formula per 24 hours, an additional 500 ml of water is required). The additional free water can be administered in two or three divided doses. The water used to flush the tube from feedings or medications should be included in this total. Tap water is fine; distilled water is unnecessary.

MONITORING

Proper monitoring of patients receiving enteral nutrition is necessary to detect and prevent complications.

1. Confirm placement of feeding tube by radiograph before initiating feeding. Studies have revealed the inaccuracy of auscultation or aspiration (23). If the feeding tube becomes dislodged, proper placement should be re-verified by radiograph.
2. Keep the patient's head and shoulders (not solely only the head of the bed) elevated at 30–458 at all times during feeding and for 1 hour after feeding is completed to prevent aspiration of the formula.
3. Use a 30–35 ml syringe to check gastric residuals every 4 hours. The residual should be , 150 ml. If not, the feeding should be held and the condition investigated. If , 150 ml, return contents to stomach. Gastric residuals may be difficult to obtain if small bore nasogastric tubes are used because the negative suction induced by the syringe will collapse the tube. Gastric residual may be increased due to delayed gastric emptying caused by recent administration of hypertonic medications in liquid form. After checking the gastric residual, the tube should be flushed with 30 ml of water to avoid clogging. Checking residuals is not useful for jejunal feeding because they do not accurately reflect jejunal emptying. Avoid the use of syringes , 30 ml because injection force when returning the residual may be sufficient to rupture the tube and cause tissue damage.
4. Maintain accurate intake and output records and record the amount of prescribed feeding actually received.
5. Record patient's weight at least three times weekly.
6. Observe the patient for abdominal distention, pain, diarrhea or dyspnea and treat accordingly.

Monitor the patient's response to therapy at least:

Every 8 hours	Vital signs
Twice weekly	Electrolytes including magnesium, calcium, phosphate, blood glucose, BUN, creatinine
Biweekly	Total protein, albumin, prealbumin, CBC with differential, AST, ALT

Monitoring frequency may be decreased in stable, long-term enterally fed patients (Fig. 4.1).

COMPLICATIONS OF ENTERAL FEEDING

Mechanical

Obstruction of the Tube Lumen

Flush the tube with 30 ml of water every 4–6 hours, after discontinuing enteral feeding and following the administration of medications through the tube to prevent any clogging of the feeding tube. Some medications are not compatible with enteral feeding and will lead to precipitation in the tube. Sucralfate should never be administered through a nasogastric feeding tube.

Adult Enteral Nutrition Orders

Baylor College of Medicine 6550 Fannin, Houston, TX 77030

Use Ball Point Pen - Press Firmly

Check Box: ☐ **Initiation Order** ☐ **Rate change only ______ mL/hr** ☐ **New Order**

ESTIMATED NEEDS	**Height ____ Current Weight ____ kg Ideal Body Weight ___ kg** Estimated caloric requirement __________ kcal/day Estimated protein requirement __________ kcal/day ☐ **Check box** to order **Indirect Calorimetry** to determine resting energy expenditure
ROUTE OF ADMINISTRATION	**Check one box:** ☐ Nasoenteric ☐ Gastrostomy ☐ Jejunostomy

FORMULA

	ISOTONIC (Osmolite)	**ISOTONIC HN (Osmolite HN)**	**ISOTONIC HIGH FIBER (Jevity)**	**CONCENTRATED (Two Cal HN)**
non-protein kcal/ml	0.91	0.89	0.93	1.69
kcal/ml	1.06	1.06	1.06	2.01
total protein g/L	36	44.4	44.5	83.4
	HIGH FAT/LOW CARB (Pulmocare)	**HYDROLYZED PROTEIN (ELEMENTAL) (Vital HN)**	**FREE AMINO ACID (ELEMENTAL) (Vivonex)**	**HIGH FIBER HIGH FAT/LOW CARB (Glucerna)**
non-protein kcal/ml	1.26	0.64	0.85	0.89
kcal/ml	1.5	1.0	1.0	1.0
total protein g/L	62.6	41.7	38.2	41.8
	Renal (Suplena)	**Renal (dialysis) (Nepro)**	**Hepatic Failure (Nutrihep)**	
non-protein kcal/ml	1.88	1.72	1.35	
kcal/ml	2.0	2.0	1.5	
total protein g/L	29.9	69.6	40	

☐ Other Nutrient Components — Check box and complete if necessary:

DIRECTIONS, INFUSING RATE, AND MONITORING

Administration method: (circle A or B). Fill in blanks.

A. **Continuous Administration**

1) Confirm tube position by x-ray before tube is used (upper abdominal x-ray for tube placement)
2) Initiate half/full **(circle one)** strength at ________ mL/hr.
3) Check gastric residuals q.4h. If residual >150 ml, hold feeding and notify M.D.
4) Elevate patient's head & shoulders 30-45E at all times during feeding & for 60 minutes after feeding is stopped.
5) Advance feeding by _____ ml every ____ hrs to a goal rate of _____ mL/hr. Once goal rate is achieved, advance to full strength after _____ hrs (does not apply to isotonic or jejunal feeding).
6) Do not stop feeding for postural drainage if patient has an endotracheal or tracheostomy tube in place with an inflated cuff.
7) Rinse feeding tube with 30 ml tap water q.4h.

B. **Cyclic or Bolus Administration** (bolus administration not recommended for J-tube feeding)

1) Confirm tube position by x-ray before tube is used (nasoenteric feeding only).
2) Gravity drop at half/full (circle one) strength feeding, ____ ml over 30 minutes q.____ hrs.
3) Check gastric residual prior to each feeding. If residual >150 ml, hold feeding and notify M.D. Do not check residuals for duodenal or jejunostomy feeding. Signs of intolerance may include nausea, vomiting, abdominal pain or distention, diarrhea.
4) Keep patient's head and shoulders elevated 30-45E at all times during feeding and for 60 minutes after feeding is stopped.
5) Rinse feeding tube with 30 ml tap water after each feeding.

The following will be performed unless otherwise ordered:
Nutrition panel I (electrolytes, glucose, BUN, creat, Ca, Mg, P) qOD x3 then q.Mon.
Nutrition panel II (alb, pre-alb, total protein, LFTs) q.Mon
Weigh patient M.W.F., Daily I and O

Date/Time Written: ______________________
Time/Date Noted: ______________________
Physician Signature: ______________________
Physician (Dictation) I.D. #: ______________________

ADDRESSOGRAPH:

Figure 4.1.
Adult enteral nutrition orders.

Protocol for Treating a Clogged Feeding Tube

Attempt to flush the tube with warm water using only mild pressure to avoid rupturing the tube. Use only finger pressure on the plunger.

Unclogging Enteric Feeding Tubes

1. Sugar-free, decaffeinated soda (does not require physician order)
2. (a) Meat tenderizer (papain). Mix 1 teaspoon non-potato flake papain meat tenderizer with the smallest amount tap water required for dissolving.
   (b) Pancrease or Viokase® (pancreatic enzyme). Mix 1 crushed pancreas enzyme tablet (Amylase 30,000 units, Protease 13,000 units, and Lipase 8,000 units per tablet) with 1 crushed tablet (324 mg) sodium bicarbonate and 5 ml tap water to prepare a pancreatic solution. Allow it to sit for 5 minutes to activate enzyme.

- Check tube position, preferably by chest or abdominal x-ray.
  1. Severe lung damage can occur if the declogging solution is administered into the bronchial tree.
- Elevate the head and shoulders of the patient's bed to an upright, or at least 45° angle.
- Clear an obstructed feeding tube as soon as possible.
- Before using any solution to declog the tubing, aspirate very slowly as much liquid from the tube as possible using a 30 to 50 ml catheter tip or Luer-lock syringe.
- Instill 5 ml or more of one of the declogging solutions using a 30 to 50 mL syringe. *Water or soda should be attempted first to unclog tubes.*
  1. Clamp the tube and wait 15 minutes.
  2. Then try to aspirate or flush the tube with water.
  3. The procedure may need to be repeated (repeat steps 1–2).
  4. Meat tenderizer and pancreatic enzyme solutions may be more effective than water or soda.
     (a) Papain-containing meat tenderizer should be obtained from the pharmacy or food service.

Esophageal Complications

- Esophagitis, erosions, ulceration, stricture or mucosal bridge function.
- More common with the use of larger tubes such as Ryle's-type or Salem-sump. Avoid these types of tubes for enteral feeding.

Nasopharyngeal Complications

- Discomfort usually minor and self-limited with small-bone tubes, but short-term use of an analgesic or anesthetic lozenges may be helpful.
- Nasal erosions and sloughing of nasal cartilage may result from excessive pressure on the nasal alae and nasal cartilage. Nasoenteric tubes should be routinely changed to the opposite nares after no more than 4–6 weeks.

- If long-term enteral feeding (> 4–6 weeks) is required, a PEG or PEJ should be placed.
- Otitis media and/or sinusitis may occur because of occlusion of sinus tracts or the eustachian tube related to pressure from the nasoenteric feeding tube. All patients who have a nasoenteric tube end are connected to a ventilator should be routinely examined with an otoscope.

Rupture of Esophageal Varices

- Does not occur with the use of small bore feeding tubes.

Trachesophageal Fistula

- Usually occurs with a large bone tube and a concurrent nasotracheal or tracheostomy tube.
- Caused by pressure necrosis and erosion through the posterior trachael wall into the anterior wall of the esophagus.

Tube Misplacement

- Tube position should be verified by radiograph before initiating feeding, or should the tube become dislodged. Auscultation may not indicate if the tube has been placed in the pleural space, lung or pharynx in an unconscious patient. (23).
- The guidewire should never be replaced in a nasoenteric feeding tube still inside the patient. The wire may exit the tube in an inappropriate location and result in esophageal or sinus perforation.
- In the situation where a nasoenteric feeding tube is dislodged or removed by a disoriented patient, a nasal bridle can be used to secure the tube (24).

Complications of PEG/PEG

1. Wound infections
   - Cellulitis at tube skin exit site
   - Abdominal abscess
   - May be prevented by the use of prophylactic antibiotics, although this may be of little help (25)
   - Necrotizing fasciitis may rarely occur if an abdominal wall infection is not recognized promptly
2. Leakage around tube
   - A small amount of secretion at the skin exit site is normal; leakage may require tube replacement with a larger-sized tube
3. Bleeding from the puncture site
4. Premature removal by patient
   - May cause separation of the stomach and anterior abdominal wall if removed within 10–14 days of placement. Keep patient NPO and pe form a water-soluble contrast study to evaluate for extravasation. A gastric leak usually requires surgical repair. After 10–14 days the tube can usually be replaced percutaneously. However, the gastrocutaneous fis-

tula may often close with 24 hours. Proper position within the gastric lumen should be documented before restarting feeding.

5. Gastrocolic fistula (PEG only)
   - Rare, usually recognized a month or more after insertion
   - Usually results with PEG removal
6. Gastric outlet obstruction (PEG only)
   - Caused by tube migration
   - Occurs more frequently with foley catheter replacement tubes because there is no external skin bolster to prevent distal tube migration
7. Gastroesophageal reflux (PEG only)
   - May be related to reduced lower esophageal sphincter pressure
8. Excessive granulation tissue (at the skin site exit)
   - May be painful
   - Treated by application of siler nitrate-impregnated cue tips

PEG/PEJ Maintenance

It is important to keep the PEG site clean and dry; occlusive dressings are unnecessary and may increase bacterial contamination because of the resultant moist environment.

Skin Irritation

- Usually related to leakage of gastric contents
- May be prevented by avoiding the use of occlusive dre ssings and keeping the PEG exit site clean and dry

Gastrostomy		Jejunostomy	
Advantages	Disadvantages	Advantages	Disadvantages
Can be placed w/o surgery	Does not decrease risk of aspiration related to delayed gastric emptying	Reduces risk of aspiration in cases of delayed gastric emptying unsuccessful	Requires surgery (endoscopically placed) PEG usually in the long-term
		No risk of GE reflux may allow more immediate post-operative feeding	Cannot use bolus feedings

Gastrointestinal Complications

Sudden nausea, vomiting, or diarrhea which develops after initiation of tube feeding may be due to:

a. Improper formula temperature
b. Irregular or too rapid administration of formula

c. Bacterial contamination of the formula
   - To avoid bacterial contamination of formula it is necessary to hang formula bags no longer than 4 hours and to change the feeding bag and tubing every 24 hours. Closed systems can be hung for 24 hours.

d. Bacterial overgrowth in the bowel

e. Hyperosmolar reactions to a formula with high osmolality when hyperosmolar formulas are infused into the stomach
   - Even diets > 700mOsm can be well tolerated when infused into the stomach if infused slowly with a pump.

f. Concurrent medication.

Most diarrhea associated with enteral feeding is usually caused by concurrent antibiotics or sorbitol as part of oral solutions (26). Nearly all formulas are lactose free. Pesola et al. (27) showed hypertonic feeding (690 mOsm) infused into the stomach in postoperative head and neck cancer patients with a mean serum albumin concentration of 2.8g/dL did not necessarily result in diarrhea.

If diarrhea develops, and is presumed secondary to the enteral feeding, the rate of feeding should first be decreased until the diarrhea resolves. If readvancement of the rate is not possible, loperamide should be administered. If this is unsuccessful, paregoric (5–20 ml) can be added to each 8-hour feeding formula volume or administered as a bolus every 4 hours through the feeding tube.

Gallstones may also develop because of impaired CCK release and gallbladder dysmotility. This problem can be avoided by the use of cyclic or bolus feeding.

Pulmonary Aspiration

Transpyloric feeding tube placement does not necessarily reduce the risk of aspiration of formula into the lungs (2).

The cause for aspiration pneumonia in patients who are enterally fed that have suffered CNS insults is largely aspiration of posterior pharyngeal secretions. This cannot be prevented by head elevation and if it occurs is usually unrelated to enteral feeding.

Metabolic Complications

The most common electrolyte abnormalities encountered in patients receiving tube feeding are hypernatremia, hyponatremia, hypercalcemia, and azotemia. These complications can often be prevented by proper monitoring of fluid intake, hydration status, and adjustment of the electrolyte content of the formula. Hyperosmotic metabolic alkalosis will result if insufficient free water is provided. Complications of overfeeding and the refeeding syndrome may also occur with enteral feeding.

HOME ENTERAL FEEDING

The patient or significant other must be trained in the use of enteral feeding, nasoenteric, gastrostomy or jejunostomy feeding tubes, site care (PEG or jejunostomy), and use of an enteral feeding pump (if necessary). Sufficient time for patient training should be allowed before discharge.

References

1. Gastroenterology 1990;98:715.
2. Strong RM, Condon SC, Solinger MR, et al. Equal aspiration rates from postpylorus and intragastric-placed small-bore nasoenteric feeding tubes: a randomized, prospective study. JPEN 1992;16:59–63.
3. Kittinger JW, Sandler RS, Heizer WD. Efficiency of metoclopramide as an adjunct to duedenal placement of small-bore feeding tubes: a randomized, placebo-controlled, double-blind study. JPEN 1987;11:33–7.
4. Radiology 1987;165:727.
5. Am J Gastroenterol 1991;86:1604–1609.
6. Page CP. Needle catheter jejunostomy. Contemp Surg 1981;19:47.
7. Schattenkerk ME, Obertop H, Bruining A, et al. Early postoperative enteral feeding by a needle catheter jejunostomy after 100 esophageal resections and reconstructions for cancer. Clin Nutr 1984;3:47.
8. Ryan JA Jr, Page CP. Intrajejunal feeding: development and current status. JPEN 1984;8:187.
9. Keohane PP, Attrill H, Love M, et al. Relation between osmolatity of diet and gastrointestinal side effects of enteral nutrition. Br Med J 1984;288:678–80.
10. Rees RG, Keohane PP. Elemental diet administrered nasogastrically without starter regimens to patients with inflammatory bowel disease. JPEN 1986;10:258–62.
11. Steinhardt HS, Wolf A, Jakobr B, et al. Protein essimilation in pancreatectomized pateients: efficiency of absorption from whole versus hydrolyzed protein. Gastroenterology 1986;90:1648.
12. Gastroenterology 1974;67:586–591.
13. Vazquez JA, Morse EL, Adibi SA. Effect of starvation on amino acid and peptide transport and peptide by hydrolysis in humans. Am J Physiol 1985;294:G563-G566.
14. Koretz RL, Meyer JH. Elemental diets—facts and fantasies. Gastroenterology 1980;78:393–410.
15. Mowatt-Larssen CA, Brown RO, Wojtsysiak SL, et al. Comparison of tolerance and nutritional outcome between a peptide and a standard enteral formula in critically ill, hypoalbuminemic patients. JPEN 1992;16:20–24.
16. Silk DB. Diet formulation and choice of enteral diet. Gut 1986;27:40–6.
17. Kemen M, Homann HH, Mumme A, et al. Is intact proteim similar for postoperative enteral nutrition than hydrolyzed protein? Clin Nutr 1991;10:37S.
18. JACN 1992;11:11–16.
19. Do patients with moderately impaired gastrointestinal function requiring enteral nutrition need a predigested nitrogen source? Gut 1992;33:877–81.
20. Dobb GJ, Towler SC. Diarrhea during enteral feeding in the critically ill: a comparison of feeds with and without fiber. Intens Care Med 1990;16:252–5.
21. Comparison of dietary protein with an oral, branched chain-enriched amino acid supplement on chronic portal-systemic encephalography. Hepatology 1984;4:279–87.

22. Heitkemper ME, Martin DL, Hansen BC, et al. Rate and volume of intermittent enteral fedding. JPEN 1981;5:125–9.
23. Metheny N. Measures to test placement of nasogastric and nosintestinal feeding tubes: a review. Nurs Res 1988;37:324–9.
24. Meer JA. A new nasal bridle for securing nasenteral feeding tubes. JPEN 1989;13:331–334.
25. Jonas SK, Neimark S, Panwalker AP. Effect of antibiotic prophylaxis in percutaneous endoscopic gastrostomy. Am J Gastroenterol 1985;80:438.
26. Edes TE, Walk BE, Austin JL. Diarrhea in tube-fed patients: feeding formula not necessarily the cause. Am J Med 1990;88:91–3.
27. Pesola GR, Hogg JE, Eisssa N, et al. Hypertonic nasogastric tube feedings: do they cause diarrhea? Crit Care Med 1990;18:1378–82.

CHAPTER 5

Pediatric Nutritional Support

NUTRITION ASSESSMENT

Nutrition assessment is an integral part of the evaluation of any child, particularly those who are not growing normally or who have an acute or chronic illness. Nutritional disturbances can occur during prolonged hospitalization particularly when oral intake is suspended or limited.

History and Physical Examination

Dietary history is of primary importance.

History should include:

- A 5-day diet diary that is analyzed by a dietician is most accurate.
- Unusual dietary habits such as fad vegetarian, sport, weight loss, or lipid lowering diets.
- Any medications (Appendix 1, Table 30).
- Evidence of anorexia (nervosa)/bulimia.
- Examination of hair, skin, teeth, mucous membranes, nails, and muscle mass is very important (Appendix 1, Table 1).

Anthropometrics

Growth can be assessed either cross-sectionally by age to determine "growth distance" or longitudinally to determine "growth velocity." The time intervals between measurements that are necessary to develop valid incremental data are listed in Table 5.1.

Weight

1. Weight for age (distance) in normal children (see Appendix 2, Figs. 1–4).
2. Weight velocity in normal children (see Appendix 2, Figs. 7, 8).
3. Premature infant weight reference values (see Appendix 2, Figs. 9, 11).
4. Weight for age (distance) in Downs Syndrome (see Appendix 2, Figs. 12–15).

Table 5.1.
Minimal Time Intervals for Velocity Measurements

Measurement	Interval
Weight	7 days
Length	4 weeks
Stature	8 weeks
Head circumference	7 days (infants)
	4 weeks (< 4 years old)
Mid-arm circumference	4 weeks

Height (Length and Stature)

Most useful indicator of growth status.

1. Length is measured while recumbent, and stature and height are measured while standing.
   - ➢ Length is measured in infants up to 36 months. It is difficult to obtain accurately and requires two measurers.
   - ➢ Stature is measured in children older than 2 years. It is obtained with bare feet. Feet, buttocks, and shoulders should all touch the measuring device. Eyes should look straight ahead.
   - ➢ See Appendix 2, Figures 1 through 4 for length or stature for age in normal children.
2. Height velocity in normal children (see Appendix 2, Figs. 5, 6).
   - ➢ Height for age below the 5th percentile is suggestive of chronic malnutrition.
3. Premature infant length reference values (see Appendix 2, Figs. 9, 10).
4. Length and stature for age (distance) in Downs Syndrome (see Appendix 2, Figs. 12–15).

Weight for Height

1. Can be used to differentiate stunting from wasting.
   - ➢ Stunting—caused by genetic or endocrine factors and results in a child small for age but a body weight proportional to length.
   - ➢ Wasting—results from nutritional deprivation and body weight is depleted out of proportion to length making the weight for height ratio low.
2. Abnormal weight-for-height ratios for children:
   - ➢ Suggestive of acute malnutrition

Calculated by dividing the actual weight by the ideal weight for the child's height (as determined from the reference graphs, Appendix 2, Figures 1–4) multiplied by 100.

Under nutrition	< 90%
Severe marasmus	< 75%
(< 65% requires hospitalization)	

Overweight	>110%
Obese	>120%

3. Weight-for-height reference values for prepubescent normal children (see Appendix 2, Figs. 16–19).

Head Circumference

- Is useful until 3 years of age when head growth slows.
- Must be measured with a non-stretchable measuring tape.
- Reference values from birth to 3 years (see Appendix 2, Figs. 16–19).
- Premature infant reference values (see Appendix 2, Fig. 9).

Mid-arm Circumference

- Measured on left arm mid-way between acromion or shoulder and olecranon or elbow.
- Normal reference values for children 1 year and older (Appendix 1, Table 3).

Mid-arm Circumference to Head Circumference Ratio

- Reflects weight for height.
- Useful when apparatus for measuring weight or height is not available.
- Accurate only up to 3 years of age when head growth slows.
- Reference values shown in Figure 5.1.

Mid-arm Muscle Circumference (see Adult Section)

Triceps Skinfold Thickness (Measures Body Fat) (see Adult Section)

Indirect Calorimetry (see Adult Section)

Body Composition

a. Fat is used preferentially as an energy source during starvation and stress. Accurate measurement of total body fat would be the ideal method to assess nutritional status.

b. Many methods to measure fat and lean body mass exist but most have limited clinical application. These include:

Total body electrical conductivity (TOBEC)
Bioelectric impedance analysis
Photon and x-ray absorptiometry
Hydrodensitometry (underwater weighing)
Total body potassium (40 K counting)
Total body water (isotope dilution)
Neutron activation

c. TOBEC is the only method that has proven practical for infants and children.

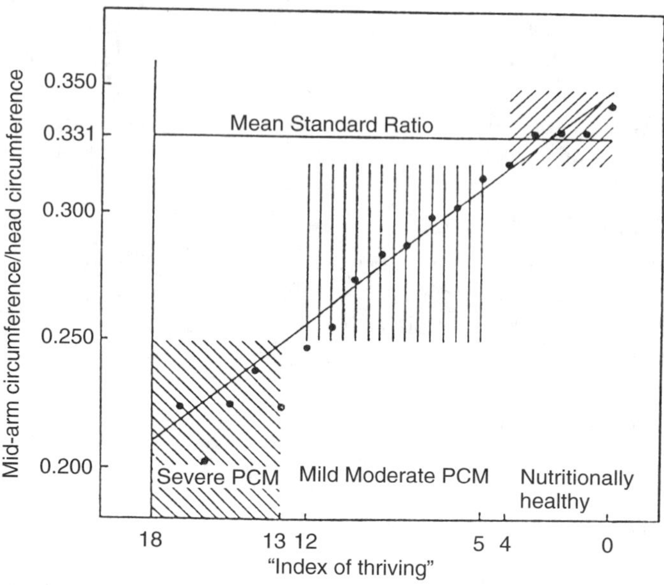

Figure 5.1.
Mid-arm circumference to head circumference ratio compared with an "index of thriving" based on weight, height, head circumference, and mid-arm circumference in PCM. Protein-calorie malnutrition. (Reprinted with permission from Kanawate A, McLaren DS. Assessment of marginal malnutrition. Nature 1970;228:573–574. Copyright 1970, Macmillan Magazines Limited.

d. The average amount of lean body mass and total body fat in non-obese normal individuals from birth to age 22 years is shown in Appendix 1, Table 6.

Laboratory Assessment

a. The initial laboratory assessment of nutritional status include the measurement of hematologic status and protein nutrition. Commonly measured serum proteins and their half-lives are listed in Table 5.2.
b. Values for protein status may not reflect the degree of nutritional deficiency since in simple starvation (marasmus) there is a tendency to maintain the circulating pool of visceral proteins at the expense of somatic protein.
c. Serum sodium and hemoglobin tend to decrease in starvation due to a dilutional effect from a physiologic increase in total body water.
d. Appendix 1, Table 30 shows normal values for some of the biochemical measurements available to evaluate nutritional status in children.
e. Immune function is reflected in total lymphocyte count and presence of anergy by skin testing.

Table 5.2.
Half Lives of Serum Proteins

Albumin	20 days
Transferrin	8 days
Prealbumin	2 days
Retinol binding protein	10 hours

NUTRITIONAL REQUIREMENTS

Fluid

Maintenance fluid requirements for children:

1600 cc per M^2 per day

To compute body surface area in M^2

$$< 5\text{ kg} = \text{kg} \times 0.05 + 0.05$$
$$5\text{–}10\text{ kg} = \text{kg} \times 0.04 + 0.1$$
$$10\text{–}20\text{ kg} = \text{kg} \times 0.03 + 0.2$$
$$> 20\text{ kg} = \text{kg} \times 0.02 + 0.3$$

Rough estimates based on body weight are as follows:

0–10 kg	100ml/kg
10–20 kg	50ml/kg
> 20 kg	20ml/kg

The fluid requirement increases by 10% for each 1°C of fever. Preterm infants have limited renal function and therefore may not tolerate fluid infusion.

Additional fluid requirements in the dehydrated child can be estimated from Table 5.3 or from actual weight loss. Composition oral electrolyte solutions are shown in the Table 5.4.

Rehydration may be accomplished orally according to methods outlined using solutions shown in Table 5.4.

Mild Dehydration

< 5%

Rehydration

ORS 40ml/kg over 4 hours.

Maintenance

Resume regular formula or lactose free formula at 150 cc/kg/day.

Replacement

ORS 10ml/kg for each diarrheal stool.

Table 5.3.
Clinical Signs of Dehydration

2–3%
Thirst, mild oliguria
5–6%
Thirst, oliguria, slightly sunken fontanel in infants, think tenacious saliva, slight decrease in skin turgor, slightly sunken eyes
7–8%
Marked thirst and oliguria, sunken fontanel, dry mouth, obvious loss of skin turgor (hypertonic dehydration causes thick doughy skin), sunken eyes with decreased intraocular tension, restlessness, or apathy
≥ 10%
As above; thirst may be lost; peripheral vasoconstriction, hypotension, cyanosis, occasional fever, increased respiratory rate (hypertonic dehydration may cause irritability and seizures)

Table 5.4.
Oral Electrolytes

	kcal/30ml	Na	K (mEq/l)	Cl	mOsm/kg H_2O	Glucose gm%
Pedialyte® (maintenance solution) (Ross)	3	45	20	35	390	2.5
Rehydralyte® (rehydration formula) (Ross)	3	75	20	65	390	2.5
Ricelyte® (maintenance solution) (Mead Johnson)	3.8	50	25	45	200	3

Moderate Dehydration

6–10%

Rehydration

ORS 100ml/kg over 4 hours.

Maintenance

Resume a lactose free formula or (1/2 strength) formula diluted 1:1 with water (for only 12–24 hr) at 150 ml/kg/day.

Replacement

ORS 10 ml/kg for each diarrheal stool.

Calories

a. Energy requirements per unit body weight are highest during the neonatal period and decline progressively until adult age.

b. Figure 5.2 shows the average caloric requirements throughout childhood. These represent averages only and should be thought of as a place to start. Individual children may require more or less energy depending on many factors such as activity, body composition, disease state, etc.

➢ The low birthweight infant may require 150 kcal/kg while normal birthweight infants require 100–120 kcal/kg.

➢ Glucose metabolism may be limited in the preterm infant. Glucose intolerance improves with age (1).

<u>Simplified Formula for Calculating Caloric Requirements in the Non-Stressed Child</u>

0–10 kg	100–115 kcal/kg	(60–80 kcal/kg for maintenance + 20 kcal/kg to support intrauterine growth rates)
11–20 kg	1000 kcal + 10 kcal/kg for each kg > 10 kg	
> 20 kg		1500 kcal + 20 kcal/kg for each kg > 20 kg

Caloric Requirements in the Stressed Child

Requirements under stress (cal/kg/day)	=	Maintenance requirements as determined	×	Conversion factor (CF) from above (cal/kg/day)

Protein

➢ Protein requirements correlate with a child's rate of growth and are highest at birth.

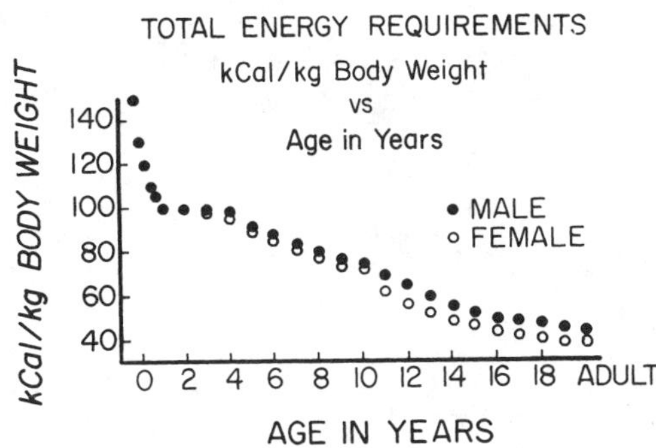

Figure 5.2.
Average caloric requirements throughout childhood.

Table 5.5.

Stress	Conversion Factor
Major surgery	1.2
Sepsis	1.2
Trauma	1.4
Burns	
< 40%	1.5
> 40%	2.0

- Figure 5.3 shows the minimal protein intake in children. Intakes up to two times that shown in the figure can be given safely. However, feeding above this increases the urea load to the kidneys and may exceed a child's excretory capacity for urea (2). Feeding less protein than is shown in Figure 5.3 can lead to protein malnutrition.
- Pre-term infants should usually be started at 1g/kg/day and advanced by 0.5–1 g/kg/day up to a maximum of 3.0–3.5 g/kg/day (3–5). Children 1–12 months old require 2.0–2.5 g/kg/day; 1.5–2g/kg/day for children 1–8 years old, and 1–1.5 g/kg/day after age 8 (3).

Electrolytes, Vitamins, Minerals, and Trace Elements

Appendix 1, Tables 10, 11, 12, and 13 show the guidelines for the use of vitamins, electrolytes, and mineral supplements in healthy infants and children. Children recovering from a nutritional insult should receive vitamin supplements. Intravenous vitamin recommendations are found in Appendix 1, Table 19.

- Fetal calcium and phosphorus accretion are approximately 130 mg/kg/day and 75 mg/kg/day, respectively (6).
- Iron supplementation is unnecessary before 2 months postnatal age. However, fetal iron accretion rates of 1000 μg/kg/day and even 200 μg/kg/day, in addition to blood transfusions, may be insufficient (7). Term infants should receive 100 μg/kg/day and preterm infants 200 μm/kg/day (8).

Table 5.6 shows the recent guidelines for the use of fluoride supplements in normal children.

PARENTERAL NUTRITION

Indications

Similar to adults (see Adult Section). In addition, short bowel syndrome may result from congenital intestinal atresia, volvulus, intussusception, gastroschisis, omphalocele, necrotizing enterocolitis, vascular infarction, and small bowel aganglionosis related to Hirshsprung's disease. Parenteral nutrition may also be required in infants with congenital villus hypoplasia and severe small in-

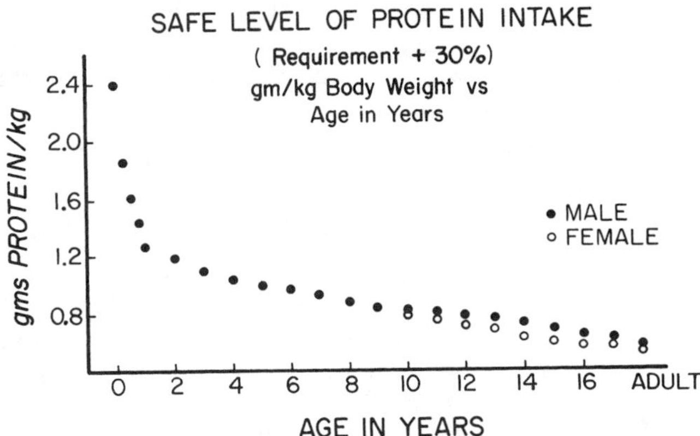

Figure 5.3.
Minimum safe levels of protein intake in children.

Table 5.6.
Flouride Supplementation

Age	Water Fluoride Content in ppm		
	< 0.3	0.3–0.6	> 0.6
Birth–6 mo	0	0	0
6 mo–3 yr	0.25	0	0
3 yr–6 yr	0.50	0.25	0
6 yr–16 yr	1.00	0.50	0

testinal mucosal damage related to protein intolerance or infection, or chronic intestinal pseudoobstruction syndrome.

- Preterm infants may have difficulty tolerating enteral feeding during the first few days or weeks after birth. For these neonates, parenteral nutrition may serve to supplement enteral feeding while slowly advancing the latter.

Peripheral Parenteral Nutrition

Dextrose concentrations ≤ 12.5%

- Starting volume should meet maintenance IV fluid requirements.
- For premature infants, increase over 12–24 hours to reach the desired rate of infusion (Table 5.7). This will achieve a caloric distribution of 8–10% protein and 50–55% carbohydrate. The remaining calories to be provided by IV fat emulsion.
- In premature infants, optimal caloric intake is difficult to reach due to fluid restriction (approx. 130 ml/kg/day).
- A scalp vein is usually used for infusion in infants < 10 kg.

Table 5.7.
Recommended Parenteral Energy Intakes

Weight (kg)	Energy (kcal/kg/day)
3–12	90–110
12–25	85–90
25–35	70–80
35–50	50–65
> 50	40

- ➢ Parenteral nutrition solutions are hyperosmolar and infiltrates can be caustic.
- ➢ Recommended solutions are shown in Appendix 1, Table 31.

Central Parenteral Nutrition

Dextrose concentrations > 15%

- ➢ Start with peripheral strength using above guidelines.
- ➢ Advance glucose concentration every 24 hours up to a maximum of 25%. For infants less than 3 months, glucose concentration should be advanced by 2.5% every 24 hours. Glucose should be monitored via serum or urine checks at least daily except (premature neonates usually stay at peripheral strength).
- ➢ See Adult Section for catheter care and management guidelines
- ➢ Solutions recommended are shown on Appendix 1, Table 32.
- ➢ Physical and occupational therapy are recommended to maintain oral motor development and feeding skills if long-term (> 2 weeks) TPN is being used.

Components of Parenteral Nutrition Solutions

Calories

Patients who are malnourished require additional calories and those with fluid losses require adjustments in mineral intake.

Calculations for Desired Rate of Infusion

1. Determine kcal per ml of TPN solution and kcal per ml of the fat solution to be used (Appendix 1, Table 20), and the kcal per kg needed (Appendix 1, Table 21).
2. Approximately 70% of calories to be supplied by the TPN solution (kcal/kg/day × .7 = calories per kg supplied by TPN).
3. Approximately 30% of calories to be supplied by the fat solution (kcal/kg/day × .3 = calories per kg supplied by fat).
4. Infusion rates:
   kg × (kcal/kg × .7) ÷ 24 hr = TPN solution, ml per hr
   TPN solution (kcal/ml)

   kg × (kcal/kg × .3) ÷ 24 hr = FAT solution, ml per hr
   FAT solution (kcal/ml)

Protein (Amino Acids)

- Cysteine may be added to neonate/infant TPN solutions at a dose of 30 mg/g amino acid to increase the solubility of calcium and phosphorus. Cysteine may be essential in neonates because of the absence of cystathionase, which converts methionine to cysteine (9). Tyrosine and histidine may also be essential for neonates.
- Taurine is contained in the neonatal amino acid solution (Trophamine®). It is an essential amino acid in these patients because of delayed cystathionase and cysteine sulfinic acid decarboxylase maturation. Taurine deficiency may lead to retinal abnormalities (10).
- Neonatal amino acid solutions contain additional tyrosine and histidine because of the limited synthetic capacity of the neonate.
- Neonatal amino acid solutions contain a lower phenylalanine concentration because excessive doses of this amino acid are associated with neurotoxicity in preterm infants (11).
- Amino acid solutions for pediatric use are based on the concentration necessary to maintain a plasma amino acid profile similar to breast milk.
- Carnitine can be added to neonatal or premature TPN solution at 8 mgm/100 cc to deboil approximately 10 mgm/kg/day.

IV Fat Emulsion

- Optimally, fat should provide 30–40% of total caloric intake. It should not exceed 60% of the total daily calorie intake.
- IV fat emulsion can be started simultaneously with the dextrose/amino acid solution, except during the first week after birth when IV fat emulsion usually is initiated 2–3 days after dextrose-amino acid solutions.
- Essential fatty acid deficiency may develop within 1–2 days in pre-term infants with absence of lipid infusion because of their limited fat stores (12).
- Administer by continuous infusion over 24 hours.
- Begin with a 20% solution at 5 ml/kg/day, which equals 1 g/kg/day or 10 kcal/kg/day.
- Advance daily by 5ml/kg to a maximum of 20 ml/kg/day, which equals 4 g/kg/day or 40 kcal/kg/day.
- Pre-term infants may have a decreased ability to clear the lipid emulsion from the blood stream and therefore, initiation should begin at 0.5 g/kg/day and be increased by 0.25–0.5 g/kg/day. Rate should not exceed 0.15 g/kg/hr. Lipid emulsions may also increase the risk of kernicterus in jaundiced neonates because the free fatty acids released during hydrolysis of the lipid compete with bilirubin for albumin binding (13).
- Serum triglycerides should be monitored with every change in lipid infusion.

Electrolytes

- IV electrolyte requirements are found in Appendix 1, Table 10.
- Acid-base abnormalities may be corrected with Na or K acetate. It is usually never given at concentrations greater than 3 mmol/dL. Acetate, a bicarbonate precursor, is soluble and stable in parenteral nutrition solutions.

Sodium bicarbonate is contraindicated because it will result in calcium/phosphorus precipitation.

- Potassium or sodium phosphate may be used to provide phosphorus.
- Calcium/phosphorus solubility in TPN solutions depends on pH, temperature, amino acid concentration, and the amino acid mixture used. The TPN dietitian or pharmacist should be contacted regarding the compatibility of calcium and phosphorus concentrations if they differ from the standard TPN protocol.

Vitamins

- Infants < 2.5 kg receive MVI-Pediatric® 2ml/kg/day.
- Infants > 2.5 kg to 11 yr: 1 vial (5 ml) MVI-Pediatric® per day.
  *Use**: MVI-pediatric® contains vitamin K, therefore additional supplementation is not necessary
- Adolescents—1 vial (10 ml) MVI-12® + Vitamin K 200 μg per day.
- Concentration of individual vitamins in standard vitamin preparations are shown in Appendix 1, Table 26.

Minerals and Trace Elements

- The pharmacy should add the appropriate amounts to meet recommendations shown in Table 5.8.
- Patients with gastrointestinal losses, renal failure, or other special situations may have different requirements.
- Iron will need to be provided if the patient is NPO longer than 2 months or enteral intake does not meet requirements.

Additives

- Insulin may be added to control blood glucose. Use 0.5–2.0 units of regular insulin per 10 grams of dextrose.
- Heparin (1 unit/ml) can be added to the solution to reduce the incidence of thrombophlebitis and preserve the patency of the line.
- Medication compatibility with parenteral nutrition is shown in Appendix 1,

Table 5.8.
Electrolyte and Trace Element Requirements

	Ca (mg/dL)	Mg (mg/L)	P (mg/L)		Zn	Cu	Cr	Mn	Se
Preterm infants	500–600	50–70	400–450	Infants < 2.5kg (μg/kg/d)	400	40	0.4	10	2
Term infants	500–600	50–70	400–450	Infants > 2.5kg (μg/kg/d)	100	10	0.1	2.5	1.5
Children	200–400	20–40	150–300	Adolescents (μg per day)	4000	1600	16	400	80

Tables 28 and 29. The use of the parenteral nutrition line for medication is to be discouraged if alternate IVs are available.

Glucose, Amino Acid, and Fat Admixtures

- In children and adolescents, the glucose/amino acid solution can be combined in one bag with IV fat emulsion (3 in 1 admixture).
- These solutions should only be used in patients whose TPN requirements are stable. They can be used in the hospital or for home patients.
- Because of potential solution instability, never alter the components or concentrations without checking with the Nutritional Support Team or pharmacy.
- Recommendations are shown in Appendix 1, Table 33.

Writing Orders

See Figure 5.4.

Monitoring Parenteral Nutrition

Complications of Parenteral Nutrition

See Adult Section.

Home TPN

a. Cycle the TPN
b. Prior to discharge
    1. Notify home health care agency 5 days before discharge.
    2. Arrange appropriate follow-up appointments for 1–2 weeks post discharge.
    3. Make arrangements for school if appropriate.
    4. Notify Occupational Therapy for instructions regarding oral stimulation and feeding skills if needed.
c. Appendix 1, Table 34 shows standard solutions for home use.
d. Laboratory monitoring
    1. If the patient's blood volume is adequate, obtain a Chem 20 and CBC weekly or every 2 weeks until stable; then every 3–4 weeks.
    2. If a Chem 20 is not available, obtain electrolytes weekly or every 2 weeks until stable, then every 3–4 weeks, ALT, AST, Alk Phos, total/direct bilirubin monthly, and calcium, phosphorus, magnesium, every 2 weeks until stable, then every 3–4 weeks.
    3. These recommendations are guidelines and may need to be individualized.
e. Daily monitoring
    1. Urine glucose twice daily, temperature daily.
f. Nutritional assessment
    1. Dietary analysis to evaluate the adequacy of nutrient intake monthly include: enteral intake, TPN, iron, and essential fatty acids.

Directions for ordering:
1. Orders should be written by 2 pm daily.
For orders received by pharmacy after hours, instead of preparing a TPN solution, the pharmacist shall prepare a stock dextrose solution with electrolytes as ordered.
2. Orders should be completely filled out.
3. Components are expressed per 100ml.
4. Mark type of TPN desired. Standard amount of TPN will be dispensed unless items marked through.

	CATHETER TYPE	
❑ Peripheral	❑ UAC/UVC	❑ single lumen
❑ Percutaneous	❑ ECMO	❑ double lumen
❑ Central	❑ Mid-line	❑ triple lumen

NURSE PLEASE COMPLETE	CASSETTE TYPE		DATE	TIME
PATIENT WEIGHT kg	TPN ❑ Micro ❑ Macro	Fat Emulsions ❑ Micro ❑ Macro	NURSE SIGNATURE	
AGE				

I. Peripheral TPN per 100ml (0.5kcal/ml)

	❑ Premature Standard	Changes	❑ Infant (0-1 year) Standard	Changes	❑ Child (1-10 years) Standard	Changes	❑ Adolescent Standard	Changes
Dextrose	12.5%		12.5%		12.5%		12.5%	
Amino Acids	2.4%		2.2%		2.2%		2.2%	
NaCl	2.6meq		2.6meq		2.6meq		4.0meq	
K_2HPO_4*	1.5mmol		1.2mmol		0.6mmol		0.5mmol	
Ca Gluconate**	1.5mmol		1.2mmol		0.5mmol		0.5mmol	
$MgSO_4$	0.5meq		0.5meq		0.8meq		1.0meq	
KCl	0.2meq		0.2meq		0.8meq		2.0meq	
Heparin	1u/ml		1u/ml		1u/ml		1u/ml	
Other								

II. Central TPN per 100ml

	❑ Premature 0.5kcal/ml Standard	Changes	❑ Infant (0-1 year) 0.5kcal/ml Standard	Changes	❑ Child (1-10 years) 0.8kcal/ml Standard	Changes	❑ Adolescent 0.8kcal/ml Standard	Changes
Dextrose	12.5%		12.5%		20.0%		20.0%	
Amino Acids	2.4%		2.2%		3.0%		3.0%	
NaCl	2.6meq		2.6meq		3.8meq		6.0meq	
K_2HPO_4*	1.5mmol		1.2mmol		1.0mmol		0.5mmol	
Ca Gluconate**	1.5mmol		1.2mmol		0.9mmol		0.5mmol	
$MgSO_4$	0.5meq		0.5meq		0.8meq		1.0meq	
KCl	0.2meq		0.2meq		1.3meq		3.0meq	
Heparin	1u/ml		1u/ml		1u/ml		1u/ml	
Other								

Added to TPN according to protocol and weight unless marked through:
Trace Minerals, Vitamins, to all TPN. L-Cysteine(30mg/gm A.A.)added to Premature/Infant TPN routinely.
Rate of Infusion ______________ ml / hour over __________ hours

III. Fat Emulsions:
❑ **20 % IV (2.0kcal/ml)** Rate of Infusion ______________ ml/hour over __________ hours

* each mmol of K_2HPO_4 contains 1.4 meq of K+ ** each mmol of Calcium Gluconate contains 2 meq Calcium Gluconate or 40 mg of elemental Calcium

IV. Comments: Additional Infusions or Piggybacks

☐ Discontinue TPN
☐ Discontinue Fat Emulsion
Date: ____/____/____

PICU DELIVERY
☐ 14:00
☐ 18:00
TIME: ____________
PAGER #: ____________

Physician Signature

ADDRESSOGRAPH

Texas Children's Hospital PHM-124 6/95

TPN-LIPID ORDER FORM

Figure 5.4.

TPN lipid order form. (Reprinted with permission from Texas Children's Hospital, Houston, Texas).

Table 5.9.
Parenteral Nutrition Monitoring Parameters

	Neonates		Beyond Neonatal Period	
	First Week	After First Week	First Week	After First Week
Strict I & O	Daily	Daily	Daily	Daily
Urine glucose	q void	q shift	q void	q shift
Electrolytes, BUN	2–3 x/wk	q wk	2–3 x/wk	q wk
Ca, PO_4, Mg, bili, Alt	q wk	q 2 wk	q wk	q 2 wk
Alk phos, albumin	-	q 2 wk	q wk	q 2 wk
Prealbumin	-	As needed	-	As needed
Serum triglycerides (TG)	See below	See below	See below	See below

Prealbumin has half-life of 2 days reflecting acute changes in protein intake; use to monitor the short term adequacy of protein intake. Serum TG: 4 hours after IV fat emulsion begun and with every increase in rate. Decrease rate if triglyceride > 150 mg/dL. Endogenous TG may be elevated during stress so pre-infusion levels suggested.

2. Infant's height, weight and head circumference should be monitored every week for the first month, then every 3–4 weeks.
3. In children, weight should be checked every 3–4 weeks.

ENTERAL NUTRITION

Transition to Enteral Feeding

- Weaning from TPN (with the exception of neonates) can usually be accomplished quickly by decreasing the rate in half 60 minutes before stopping TPN and in half again 30 minutes before stopping TPN. Neonates need to be weaned slowly over 1 to 2 days.
- When stopped, ensure that essential fatty acid needs are met enterally (4% of total calories).

Feeding Methods

Nipple Feeding

- Breast or bottle
- Attempt with infants that are at least 32 weeks of gestation age

Continuous Drip Orogastric/Nasogastric Feeding

Do not use nasogastric route in pre-term infants who are obligatory nose breathers

- Initiate with 1/2 strength formula at 1–2 ml/kg/hr, advance by 1–2 ml/kg every 8–12 hr as tolerated until fluid requirements met, then advance strength to 3/4 strength then full strength every 24 hours as tolerated (max. rate: 55 ml/hr). Check residuals every 4 hr and hold feeding if > 2x previous hourly rate volume.

- Nocturnal continuous infusion may be useful in preventing hypoglycemia in children with glycogen storage disease (15).

Intermittent Feedings

- Initiate full strength formula at 2–5 ml/kg every 3–4 hr and advance by 2–5 ml/kg every two feedings as tolerated until optimal calories achieved (16).
- Check residual prior to each feeding and hold feeding if volume > 2x previous volume infused and patient is symptomatic with abdominal distention or vomiting. Attempt refeeding in 1 hour if residual decreases.
- Less energy expenditure with continuous feeding (17).

Infant Formulas (Tables 5.10 and 5.11)

Breast feeding is optimal mode of feeding the normal term infant, but since not all infants have access to human milk, nutritious alternatives to human milk have been developed. The composition of infant formulas has evolved over the past century as our understanding of nutrient requirements, absorptive physiology, and metabolic disturbances has advanced. A large array of normal infant formulas and special purpose formulas is currently available. To select the proper formula, understand the significance of the various nutrients comprising them.

Caloric Content

Commerically prepared formulas are available as:

- Concentrated liquid containing 40 calories per 30 ml
- Powder containing approximately 40 calories per tablespoon
- Liquid ready-to-feed containing 20 calories per 30 ml

Whole cow milk and human milk both contain approximately 20 calories per ounce (.67 calories per ml). This is the standard caloric density for formula

Table 5.10.
Examples of Various Infant Formulas

Concentrated Liquids	Ready-to-Feed	Powder
Isomil	Similac 20, 24 & 27	Enfamil Human Milk Fortifier
Similac	Similac Natural Care 24	Pregestimil
Enfamil	Similac Special Care 20 & 24	Portagen
Prosobee	Similac PM 60/40	Similac PM 60/40
Nursoy	Enfamil Premature 20 & 24	Product 3232A
Soyalac	Alimentum	Product 80056
RCF	Nutramigen	S-29
SMA	Good Start	ProViMin
I-Soyalac	Enfamil 20 & 24	Nutramigen
	Isomil 20	Gerber
	Prosobee 20	
	SMA 20 & 24	
	Nursoy 20	

TABLE 5.11.
Caloric Conversions for Some Powdered Infant Formulas

Nutramigen:	4.6 kcal/gm, 9.7 gm/packed level scoop. 141 gm/packed level cup
Pregestimil:	5.0 kcal/gm, 8.8 gm/packed level scoop, 128 gm/unpacked level cup
Portagen:	4.72 kcal/gm, 7.23 gm/level unpacked scoop, 136 gm/packed level cup
Similac:	4.58 kcal/gm, 8.74 gm/level unpacked scoop, 123 gm/level unpacked cup
Similac PM 60/40:	4.65 kcal/gm, 8.6 gm/level unpacked scoop, 123 gm/level unpacked cup
Isomil:	4.55 kcal/gm, 8.79 gm/level unpacked scoop, 123 gm/level unpacked cup
Enfamil:	5.25 kcal/gm, 8.3 gm/level unpacked scoop, 121 gm/level unpacked cup
Prosobee:	5.18 kcal/gm, 8.6 gm/level unpacked scoop, 124 gm/level unpacked cup
Lofenalac:	4.6 kcal/gm, 9.6 gm/packed level scoop, 139 gm/level packed cup
Vital (Adult Formula):	79 gm/packet + 255 mL H_2O = 300 mL = 300 kcal
Product 3232A:	5.0 kcal/gm 6.3 gm/Tbsp (12.7 kcal/oz without added CHO)
Product 80056:	4.9 kcal/gm (22.5 gm fat & 78.1 gm CHO/100 gm powder) 9.05 gm/Tbsp
RCF-conc. liquid:	24 kcal/oz (12 kcal/oz diluted without added CHO)
S-29:	4.79 kcal/gm, 9.4 gm/Tbsp

preparation.There are three methods for providing a higher calorie infant formula:

- Hyper-concentrated formula:
  e.g., Prosobee 24 kcal/oz
  - Provides 20% higher protein, fat, CHO, and osmolarity
  - Beneficial because all nutrients are increased
- Add fat or carbohydrate:
  e.g. Portagen 20 + Polycose = 24 kcal/oz
- Add oil: e.g., Similac 20 + MCT oil = 24 kcal/oz
- Combination of above:
  Isomil 24 + Polycose = 27 kcal/oz + MCT oil = 30 kcal/oz
- Addition of calorie additives may "dilute" specific nutrients such as protein

Human Milk

- Human milk can be given to infants whose mothers are expressing and storing their milk.
- Human milk contains approximately 20 calories per ounce (.67 calories per ml). To increase the caloric density and the protein and mineral content of human milk for low birth weight infants, add 4 packets of Human Milk Fortifier (Mead Johnson) to each 100 cc milk.
- When initiating fortification in low birth weight infants, start with 2 packets per 100 cc for he first day and increase to 4 packets on the second day.
- Special concerns when feeding human milk by gavage: the use of continuous drip with human milk results in substantial losses of fat unless an automatic syringe pump is used, and the tip of the syringe is oriented upright to avoid loss of fat.
- Consider "hindmilk" as an energy supplement due to its high fat content.
- The composition of various milks is shown in Appendix 1, Table 35.

Milk-Based Formulas

Standard milk-based formulas normally used for routine infant feeding are shown in Appendix 1, Table 36.

Soy-Based Formulas

Composition of soy-based formulas are shown in Appendix 1, Table 37.
These formulas are indicated in infants with lactose intolerance. Some infants with allergy to cow milk protein may tolerate soy formulas but cross-reactivity may occur in these infants.

Specialized Formulas

Special infant formulas are listed in Appendix 1, Table 38.
These formulas all have specific indications for use and are not indicated in the normal infant.

Formulas Designed for Low Birth Weight Infants

Low birth weight formulas are listed in Appendix 1, Table 39.

Modular Formulas

The products listed in Appendix 1, Table 40 were developed to help treat specific nutritional problems. They are not complete diets and care should be taken to make sure the patient's total intake is adequate when using them.

Infant Formula Additives

Many nutrients are available to increase specific nutrient or calorie concentrations in infant formulas. These are listed in Appendix 1, Table 41.

Tube Feeding

Tube feedings ("milk drips") are available for both infants and children. Infant formulas are used for total or supplemental nutrition from birth to 1 year of age. Adult enteral products can be used for the pediatric patient older than 1 year of age, however, they have a higher protein and sodium content and a higher vitamin/mineral base. PediaSure is a complete enteral formula designed for children between 1–6 years.

Transition to Solid Food

Because iron stores are limited in the infant, the first solid food recommended is iron-fortified infant cereal. After this, the sequence of introduction is dictated primarily by tradition and is listed in the following table.

Month	Food Items
1–4	Breast milk or formula only
4–6	Iron-fortified cereal
6–7	Strained fruits; begin introducing cup

7–8	Strained vegetables
8–9	Start finger foods and chopped (junior food)
9	Meats, citrus juice
10	Bite-sized cooked foods
12	All table foods

Complications of Enteral Feeding

See Adult Section

REFERENCES

1. Pediatrics 1974;53:189–95.
2. Am J Dis Child 1983;135:1008–16.
3. Zlotlein SH, Bryen MH, Anderson GH. Intravenous nitrogen and energy intakes required to duplicate in utero nitrogen accretion in prematurely born human infants. J Peds 1981;99:105–120.
4. Kashyap S, Forsyth M, Zucker C, et al. Effects of varying protein and energy intakes on growth and metabolic response in low birth weight infants. J Peds 1986;108:955–963.
5. Am J Clin Nutr 1986;43:108–111.
6. Kover IZ, Morgan JB. Parenteral nutrition in the preterm infant. Clin Nutr 1990;9:57–63.
7. Sturman A, Gaull G, Raiha NCR. Absence of cystathionese in human fetal kiver: Is cystine essential? Pediatrics 1995;19:114–118.
8. Am J Clin Nutr 1988;48:1324–42.
9. Science 1970;169:74–78.
10. Biol Neonate 1977;32:73–6.
11. Lancet 1986;1105.
12. Committee on Nutrition. Iron supplementation for infants. Pediatrics 1976;58:640–9.
13. Thiessen H, Jacobsen J, Brodersen R. Displacement of albumin-bound bilirubin by fatty acids. Acta Paed Scand 1972;61:285–8.
14. Am J Clin Nutr 48:1324–1342, 1988
15. Heird WC, Driscoll JM, Schullinger JN, et al. Intravenous alimentation in pediatric patient. J Peds 1972;80:351–372.
16. Marian M. Pediatric nutrition support. Nutr Clin Pract 1993;8:199–209.
17. Grant J, Denne SC. Effect of intermittent versus continous enteral feeding on energy expenditure in premature infants. J Peds 1991;118:928–32.

CHAPTER 6

Nutritional Support During Pregnancy

Adequate nutrition during pregnancy is mandatory to ensure proper fetal development and maternal health.

- Malnutrition during pregnancy is associated with a high incidence of fetal death, prematurity, low birth weight, and decreased brain size.
- Possible indications for parenteral nutrition during pregnancy include: hyperemesis gravidarum, active Crohn's disease, or disease restricting oral intake, anorexia, cystic fibrosis, pancreatitis.
- See Appendix 1, Table 44 for laboratory changes during pregnancy.

WEIGHT GAIN

- 10% 1st trimester
- 20–30% 2nd trimester; > 0.5–1.0 lb (0.2–0.5 kg) per week
- 60% 3rd trimester
- Total = 20–25 (9–12 kg) lb
- Weight gain < 14 lb (6.5 kg) = weight loss

Targets for Weight Gain

- > 120% IBW
  → Total 3–4 kg (7–8 lb) = 300 g/wk
- IBW (patient not planning to nurse infant)
  → Total 4.5 kg (10 lb) = 350 g/wk
- IBW (will nurse infant)
  → Total 5.5 kg (12 lb) = 400 g/wk
- < 90% IBW
  → Total 6.3–6.8 kg (14–15 lb) = 500 g/wk

METABOLIC CHANGES

These should be anticipated when providing nutritional support

- Plasma glucose concentration declines
- Stimulated insulin secretion increases
- Peripheral insulin resistance

- Altered lipid metabolism with increased VLDL, total cholesterol, LDL, and HDL

NUTRITIONAL REQUIREMENTS

Calories

RDA + 300 kcal/d = 55,000 extra calories for pregnancy

- Recommendation recently questioned (1).
- Lactation: RDA + 525–745 kcal/day assuming 600–850 ml/day milk produced

Protein

RDA + 10 g/day 1st trimester, add 1.3 g/day
or
1st trimester: add 1.3 g/day
2nd Trimester add 6.1 g/day
3rd Trimester add 10.7 g/day
Lactation 1.5 g/kg/day (2)

Fat

- Extreme dietary deficiency of essential fatty acids is associated with decreased brain lipid content and impaired learning ability in newborn animals
- Monitor the serum triglyceride concentration
- Necessary for prostaglandin synthesis
- An additional 1.5% of total maternal calories should be provided as linoleic acid (3)

Minerals and Trace Elements

- For the RDA of mineral and vitamins during pregnancy and location see Appendix 1, Tables 11, 12 and 13.
- There is little data on optimal parenteral requirements.

Calcium, Magnesium

- May decline by 10–15% usually related to decreased serum albumin caused by hemodilution

Zinc

- Plasma concentration declines 20–25% beginning in the mid 1st trimester. This may also be related to decreased serum albumin.
- Deficiency may cause fetal growth retardation, multiple congenital abnormalities, particularly of the skeletal and nervous systems, and low birth weight.

Iron

- Deficiency is associated with infant anemia.

Copper

- Serum concentration increases up to 1.5–4x pregnancy, paralleling the increase in ceruloplasmin.
- Deficiency (rare) is associated with placental insufficiency and intrauterine death.

Vitamins

Niacin

- Urinary excretion of one metabolite, H-methyl nicotinamide increases during the second trimester.

Pyridoxine

- Plasma concentration decreases in the third trimester.

Vitamin B_{12}

- Plasma concentration decreases up to 1000 pg/dL throughout pregnancy.

Folate

- Decrease is most likely related to the depletion of maternal stores.
- The greatest risk of deficiency is in multigravida and in mothers receiving anticonvulsants.
- Deficiency is associated with fetal neural tube defects, toxemia of pregnancy, and premature labor.

Ascorbic Acid (Vitamin C)

- Plasma concentration decreases 10–15% but is without known consequence, although an association with premature membrane rupture has been reported.

Thiamine

- Urinary thiamine excretion increases during the 2nd and 3rd trimesters. There is no change in erythrocyte transketolase however.
- Deficiency may cause fatal heart failure in the newborn.

Riboflavin

- Urinary excretion increases during the 2nd trimester and decreases during the 3rd trimester. There is no change in erythrocyte glutathione reductase activity, however.

Vitamin A

- Serum concentration decreases during the 1st trimester, then gradually increases throughout the remainder of pregnancy.
- Megadoses (> 8000 IV/day) are associated with congenital urinary tract malformation and neural tube defects.

Vitamin D

- The serum 25-OH D3 concentration is usually unchanged during pregnancy, but deficiency may be associated with neonatal hypocalcemia and osteomalacia.

Vitamin E

- The serum concentration may increase by 40–60% beginning in the 2nd trimester.

Vitamin K

- No increase in the prothrombin time has been observed during pregnancy in the absence of fat malabsorption or bacterial overgrowth.

References

1. Mughal MM, Shaffer JL, Turner M, et al. Nutritional management of pregnancy in patients on home parenteral nutrition. Br J Obstet Gynecol 1987;94:44–9.
2. Motil KJ, Montandon CM, Thotathuchery M, et al. Dietary protein and nitrogen balance in lactating and nonlactating women. Am J Clin Nutr 1990;51:378–84.
3. Crawford MA. Estimation of essential fatty acid and requirements in pregnancy and lactation. Prog Food Nutr Sci 1980;4:75–80.

CHAPTER 7

Assessing the Efficacy of Nutritional Therapy

Nutritional goals should be established and re-evaluated at regular intervals.

DAILY INPUT AND OUTPUT RECORD

Evaluate the input and output record daily to determine what proportion of the prescribed nutritional order is actually received. Interrupted delivery of parenteral nutrition is not uncommon e.g., during blood transfusion. Intravenous pumps may often be 10% and occasionally up to 25% inaccurate. Likewise, enteral nutrition is often interrupted because of medical procedures, tube repositioning, etc.

WEIGHT

Comparison of serial weights is an easy way to assess response to nutritional therapy. If weight gain is anticipated, it should be on the order of 2–3 pounds (1–2 kg) weekly. Weight gain greater than this, especially during parenteral nutrition, is more often due to fluid retention. Physical examination and close inspection of daily inputs and outputs will help to determine if fluid retention is occurring. Often, presacral edema occurs long before pedal edema, especially in a patient lying prone in bed where the lower back and gluteal regions lie in the most dependent position.

VISCERAL PROTEINS

Prealbumin is the preferred visceral protein to assess response to nutritional therapy.

It should be checked on the fourth day of therapy. Due to its short half-life (1.9 days), an increase in serum prealbumin should be observed within the first 4–7 days. This increase is believed to correlate with increased protein synthesis and anabolism.

Because albumin has a very long half-life (21 days), it will not be responsive to short-term changes in visceral protein status and should not be monitored more often than on a weekly basis unless albumin is exogenously infused to treat hypo-oncotic edema.

Increased serum albumin related to exogenous albumin administration has no relationship to changes in nutritional status.

It may be difficult to normalize serum albumin if ongoing losses occur from severe protein losing enteropathy, wound drainage or exudate, burns, or nephrotic syndrome despite provision of nutritionally adequate therapy.

In markedly hypermetabolic patients, such as those with head trauma or spinal cord injuries, anabolism may not be achievable initially. Therefore, the initial goal should be to limit catabolism.

The role of growth factors such as growth hormone and IGF-1 are under investigation in these situations and should not be used outside of investigational protocols because of their expense, undetermined efficacy, and potential metabolic side effects.

CELLULAR IMMUNITY

Total lymphocyte count is one of the earliest indicators to show response to nutritional support. However, non-nutritional factors can obviate use of this parameter.

NITROGEN BALANCE

A negative nitrogen balance is associated with catabolism while a positive nitrogen balance is associated with net nitrogen retention and anabolism. Positive nitrogen balance greater than 4 is desirable.

Nitrogen balance can be determined after 3–4 days of nutritional support to assess the adequacy of caloric and protein provision. A positive nitrogen balance requires both sufficient protein *and* calories.

PHYSICAL EXAMINATION

Signs of specific nutrient deficiencies and nutritionally dependent processes such as wound healing and fistula closure should be monitored to show improvement and/or resolution.

MUSCLE FUNCTION

Hand grip strength or maximal inspiratory/expiratory pressure can be followed. Skeletal muscle strength can be measured using handgrip dynamometry (1, 2), or maximal inspiratory or expiratory force (3). Both are excellent methods of assessment, but require patient cooperation, which may be impossible in a physically disabled or ventilated patient, respectively.

DRUG-NUTRIENT INTERACTION

Certain nutrient deficiencies may occur during treatment despite the provision of a usual maintenance dose of the nutrient in question. See Appendix 1, Table

30 for potential drug-nutrient interactions, which may require additional supplementation of some nutrients.

References

1. Klidjian AM, Foster KJ, Kammerling RM. Relation of anthropometric and dynamometric variables to serious postoperative complications. Br Med J 1980;281:899–901.
2. Hunt DR, Rowlands BJ, Johnston D. Hand grip strength—a simple prognostic indicator in surgical patients. JPEN 1985;9:701–4.
3. Kelly SM, Rose A, Field S. Inspiratory muscle strength and body composition in patients receiving total parenteral nutrition therapy. Am Rev Respir Dis 1984;130:33–7.

CHAPTER 8

Disease-Specific Nutrition

ACUTE RENAL FAILURE

Restrict protein intake to 0.8 g/kg/day in non-dialyzed patients. Patients fed 0.6–0.7 g/kg/day become protein malnourished and have a poorer outcome. There is a theoretical advantage to using formulas containing only essential amino acids, but no proven clinical efficacy (1,2). These formulations are also substantially more expensive than standard amino acid solutions. Provide 35 kcal/kg/day or use indirect calorimetry. Monitor fluid load, serum potassium, and phosphate closely. Renal failure specific formulas such as AminAid®, Suplena®, or Nepro® may be useful in patients with hyperkalemia, hypermagnesemia, or hyperphosphatemia with standard products. There is no demonstrated benefit with respect to morbidity or mortality with these products, however.

CHRONIC RENAL FAILURE (OR ARF WITH DIALYSIS)

Protein intake should not be restricted, but increased to account for amino acid loss in the dialysate. This amounts to 6–8 g in hemodialysis, 12–16 g during peritoneal dialysis, and 12–16 g/day for continuous hemofiltration (3). The amino acid histidine is considered essential in renal failure. Water soluble vitamin deficiency can occur, most especially pyridoxine (B_6) because these vitamins are removed in the dialysate. In contrast, fat soluble vitamins are not removed. Vitamin E is essentially nontoxic and 1,25 dihydroxy-vitamin D concentration is likely to be low on the basis of decreased α-hydroxylation in the kidney. Vitamin A accumulation and toxicity may, however, be a concern. Provide 35 kcal/kg/day or use indirect calorimetry. Patients with chronic renal failure may exhibit fat intolerance and, therefore, the serum triglyceride concentration should be followed carefully to ascertain adequate clearance of lipid emulsion.

RESPIRATORY FAILURE

Care should be taken to avoid overfeeding. Overfeeding may result in increased CO_2 production, which will impede successful ventilator weaning. Avoiding overfeeding is far more important and much less expensive than specialty pulmonary formulas. Pulmocare® provides a greater percentage of calories as lipid than dextrose. Theoretically, its metabolism should produce less CO_2. Clinically, the effects on CO_2 production differ little from standard, higher carbohydrate-containing formulas. The use of Pulmocare® should be reserved for the marginal patient only. This is the only product in this category for which published clinical data currently exists. The caloric requirements for a nonventilated patient with COPD may be difficult to estimate. Unlike nutritionally depleted patients without lung disease who may lose 10% or more of their body weight and who have a measured REE less than predicted, patients with similar degrees of weight loss may have a 10–25% increase in REE due to the work of breathing (4). Failure to provide adequate nutrition will eventually result in a reduction in respiratory muscle strength (5), hypoxic ventilatory drive (6), and minute ventilation (6, 7). The margin between underfeeding and overfeeding in this patient group may be small and the use of indirect calorimetry is probably prudent. Patients with marginal respiratory function also should not receive excessive amino acids because high nitrogen intake increases the threshold response to CO_2. The serum phosphate concentration should be monitored specifically, as severe hypophosphatemia may lead to prolonged respiratory failure because of skeletal muscle dysfunction and impaired diaphragm contractility (8–10). Patients with ARDS may experience a transient decrease in PaO_2 during lipid emulsion infusion (11).

HEPATIC FAILURE

See discussion of branched chain amino acids.

REFERENCES

1. Leonard CD, Luke RG, Siegel RR. Parenteral essential amino acids in acute renal failure. Urology 1975;6:154–7.
2. Feinstein EI, Blumenkrantz. Clinical and metabloic responses to parenteral nutrition in acute renal failure: a controlled double-blind study. Medicine 1981;60:124–37.
3. Frankenfield DC, Badellino MM, Reynolds HN. Amino acids loss and plasma concentration during continuous hemodiafiltration. JPEN 1993;17:551–61.
4. Goldstein S, Askanazi J, Thomashaw B, et al. Metabolic demand, ventilation and muscle function during repletion of malnourished COPD and surgical patients. Anesthesiology 1985;63:A276.
5. Arora NS, Rochester DF. Respiratory muscle strength and maximal voluntary ventilation in undernourished patients. Am Rev Resp Dis 1982;126:5–8.
6. Doekel RC, Zwillich CW, Scoggin CH, et al. Clinical semi-starvation: depression of hypoxic ventilatory response. N Engl J Med 1979;295:358–361.
7. Weissman C, Askanazi J, Rosenbaum S, et al. Amino acids and respiration. Ann Intern Med 1983;98:41–4.
8. N Engl J Med 1977;296:1101–3.

9. Aubier M, Murciano D, Lecocguic Y. Effect of hypophosphatemia on diaphragmatic contractility in patients with acute respiratory failure. N Engl J Med 1985;313:420–4.
10. Grevelyn TR, Brophy N, Siegert C, et al. Hypophosphatemia-associated respiratory muscle weakness in a general inpatient population. Int J Surg 1982;67:371–2.
11. Crit Care Med 1984;12:293.

APPENDIX 1

Tables

Table 1.
Clinical Signs of Nutrient Deficiencies

Clinical Finding	Consider Deficiency	Comment
Hair		
Easily pluckable, sparse	Protein, biotin, zinc	Loss of scalp and body hair may also occur
Straight, dull	Protein	Hair will be fine and silky
Flag sign	Protein, copper	Reddening of normally black scalp; occurs in black-skinned children, possibly due to abnormal sebaceous gland activity
Coiled-corkscrew-like	Vitamin A, C	Due to follicular change; due to a keratinization disturbance and possibly abnormal sebaceous gland activity
Skin		
Xerosis	Essential fatty acid	Dryness of skin
Petechiae	Vitamin A, vitamin C	Pin-headed sized hemorrhages
Pigmentation Desquamation	Niacin	Signs of pellagra distributed symmetrically in sun-exposed areas; also seen in hemochromatosis, an iron storage disease
Follicular hyperkeratosis	Vitamin A, possibly essentially fatty acid deficiency	Keratin plugs in follicles, sandpaper feel of skin
"Flakey-pain" dermatitis	Protein	
Subcutaneous fat loss, fine wrinkling	Protein-energy	Minimal fat reserves; low values for anthropometric indices
Poor tissue turgor	Water	
Edema	Protein, thiamine	Seen in protein-energy malnutrition with hypoalbuminemia and in wet beriberi due to thiamine deficiency
Purpura (subcutaneous skin hemorrhage)	Vitamin C, vitamin K	
perifollicular hemorrhage	Vitamin C	
Pallor	Folate, iron, B12, copper	
Excessive hair growth	Protein-energy	Like fetal lanugo; noticeable in girls with anorexia nervosa; may be heat-retaining mechanism
Tendency toward excessive bruising (ecchymoses)	Vitamin C, vitamin K	Due to increased fragility of capillary walls
Pressure sores	Protein-energy	Common in pressure and bony points
Seborrheic dermatitis	Essential fatty acid, pyridoxine, Zinc	Also seen in acrodermatitis enteropathica due to a defect in zinc absorption

Table 1. (*continued*)
Clinical Signs of Nutrient Deficiencies

Clinical Finding	Consider Deficiency	Comment
Poor wound healing	Protein-energy, zinc, and possibly essential fatty acids	Scrotal or vulvar in riboflavin deficiency; nasolabial in pyridoxine deficiency
Dermatitis	Biotin	
Dry scaling	Nonspecific	
Thickening of skin	Essential fatty acid	
Eyes		
Angular palpebritis	Riboflavin	Can lead to xerophthalmia in severe deficiency
Dull, dry conjunctiva (xerosis)	Vitamin A	Angular in riboflavin deficiency
Blepharitis	B vitamins	Wernicke's syndrome; prompt treatment necessary
Ophthalmoplegia	Thiamine	Softening of cornea
Keratomalacia	Vitamin A	Early evidence of deficiency
Bitot's spot	Vitamin A	
Corneal vascularization	Riboflavin	
Photophobia	Zinc	
Lips and Oral Structures		
Angular fissures, scars, or stomatitis	B-vitamins, iron, protein, riboflavin	Also seen with ill-fitting dentures Seen especially at corners of mouth
Cheilosis	B-6, niacin, riboflavin, protein	Also associated with altered sense of smell
Dysgeusia	Zinc	If not edentulous
Swollen, spongy, bleeding gums	Ascorbic acid	
Tongue		
Magenta tongue	Riboflavin	Controversial; magenta color may also be due to poor general nutrition
Fissuring, raw	Niacin	Due to inadequate repair of epithelial tissues
Glossitis		
Large size, swollen	Iodine, niacin	In niacin deficiency, the tongue can be deeply fissured
Fiery red tongue	Folate, B_{12}	Seen if anemia is not pronounced
Atrophic lingual papillae	Riboflavin, niacin	
Teeth		
Loss of dental fillings, dental caries	Vitamin C	Scurvy

Table 1. (*continued*)
Clinical Signs of Nutrient Deficiencies

Clinical Finding	Consider Deficiency	Comment
Glands		
Parotid enlargement	Protein	Rate, seen in alcoholic patients
Thyroid enlargement	Iodine	Seen in areas where deficiency has not been corrected by table salt iodination
Hypogonadism, delayed puberty	Zinc	
Nails		
Spoon-shaped nails (koilonychia)	Iron	
Brittle, ridged, lined nails	Protein-energy	May be protein undernutrition
Heart		
Tachycardia, cardiomegaly, congestive heart failure	Thiamine (wetberi-bers)	"Wet" beriberi associated with high output congestive heart failure
Decreased cardiac function	Phosphorous	
Cardiac arrhythmias	Magnesium, potassium	
Cardiomyopathy	Selenium, copper	Referred to as Keshan disease in the Orient. Occurrence in the U.S. with parenteral nutrition
Small heart, decreased output, bradycardia	Protein-energy	Prone to congestive heart failure during refeeding
Sudden failure, death	Ascorbic acid, thiamine	In ascorbic acid deficiency, death may be due to myocardium hemorrhage
Abdomen		
Hepatomegaly (fatty liver)	Protein, fatty acid	Also commonly seen in alcoholics
Wasting	Energy	Found in marasmus
Bones and Joints		
Bone pain	Calcium, vitamin D, phosphorous, vitamin C	Osteomalacia due to repeated pregnancies with poor Ca intake, little sunlight, steatorrhea
Muscles, Extremities		
Wasting	Protein-energy	Evidence in temporal area, dorsum of hand between thumb and index fingers, calf muscles
Edema	Protein	
Muscular twitching	Protein, thiamine selenium	
Muscular pain	Sodium, potassium	
Muscle cramps	Sodium, chloride	

Table 1. (*continued*)
Clinical Signs of Nutrient Deficiencies

Clinical Finding	Consider Deficiency	Comment
Neurologic		
Ophthalmoplegia, footdrop	Thiamine	Wernicke's encephalopathy
Disorientation	Thiamine, sodium, water	Korsakoff's psychosis; confabulation occurs in thiamin-deficient alcoholics
Decreased position, vibratory sense, ataxia, optic neuritis	B_{12}	Subacute combined cord degeneration
Weakness, paresthesia of legs	Thiamine, pyridoxine, pantothenic acid, B_{12}	Nutritional polyneuropathy, especially with alcoholism; "burning foot" syndrome with pantothenic acid deficiency
Hyporeflexia	Thiamin	
Mental disorders	Niacin, B_{12}	In untreated B_{12} deficiency, mental disorders may progress to severe psychosis
Convulsions	Pyridoxine, calcium, thiamine (infants), magnesium, phosphorous	
Depression, lethargy	Biotin, vitamin C	
Nonketonic hyperosmolar syndrome	fluid	
Hyperesthesia		Due to large glucose infusions that result in an osmotic diuresis; occurs in TPN patients
Peripheral neuropathy	Sodium Pyridoxine, vitamin E	
Other		
Diarrhea	Niacin	
Delayed wound healing and tissue repair	Vitamin C, zinc, protein-energy zinc, fatty acid	
Anemia, pallor	pyridoxine, B_{12}, iron, folate, copper	
Anorexia	B_{12}, sodium, thiamine, vitamin C	
Fatigue, lassitude, apathy	Energy, biotin, magnesium, phosphorous, iron, potassium, sodium	
Growth retardation	Protein-energy, magnesium, zinc, vitamin D, calcium	
Constipation	Thiamine	GI dysmotility
Glucose intolerance	Chromium?	
Bleeding diathesis	Vitamin K	

Table 2.
Metropolitan Life Weight Chart (1983)

Height		Men (kg)			Women (kg)		
Inches	Cm	Small frame	Medium frame	Large frame	Small frame	Medium frame	Large frame
58	147				46–50	46–55	54–60
59	150				47–51	50–60	55–61
60	152				47–52	51–57	55–62
61	155				48–54	52–59	57–63
62	157	58–61	60–64	62.7–68.2	49–55	54–60	58–65
63	160	59–61.8	60.4–65	63–69.5	50–56	55–61	60–69
64	163	60–62.7	61.3–65.9	64.5–71	52–58	56–63	61–69
65	165	60.9–63	62.2–67.2	65.4–72.7	53–59	58–64	62–70
66	168	61.8–64.5	63.2–68.6	66–74.5	55–60	59–65	63–72
67	170	62.7–65.9	64.5–70	67.7–76.3	56–62	60–67	65–74
68	172	63–67.3	65.9–71.3	69–78	56–62	62–68	66–80
69	173	64.5–68.6	67.3–72.7	70.4–80	57–63	69–70	68–77
70	178	65.4–70	68.6–74	71.8–81.8	58.6–64.5	64–71	69–79
71	180	66–71.3	70–75.4	73.2–83.6	60–65.9	66–72	70–80
72	183	67.7–72.7	71.3–77.2	74.5–85.4	61–67	67–74	72–81
73	185	69–74.3	73–79	76–87	63–69		
74	188	70.4–76.3	74.5–80.9	78–89.5			
75	191	71.8–78	75.9–83	80–92			
76	193	73.6–80	78–85	82–94			

Table 3.
Arm Measurements

Percentiles of Upper Arm Circumference (mm) and Estimated Upper Arm Muscle Circumference (mm) for Whites of the United States Health Examination Survey 1 of 1971 to 1974

	Arm Circumference (mm)						Arm Muscle Circumference (mm)					
	5th	50th	95th	5th	50th	95th	5th	50th	95th	5th	50th	95th
Age (yr)	Males			Females			Males			Females		
1–1.9	142	159	183	138	156	177	110	127	147	105	124	143
2–2.9	141	162	185	142	160	184	111	130	150	111	126	147
3–3.9	150	167	190	143	167	189	117	137	153	113	132	152
4–4.9	149	171	192	149	169	191	123	141	159	115	136	157
5–5.9	153	175	204	153	175	211	128	147	169	125	142	165
6–6.9	155	179	228	156	176	211	131	151	177	130	145	171
7–7.9	162	187	230	164	183	231	137	160	190	129	151	176
8–8.9	162	190	245	168	195	261	140	162	178	138	160	194
9–9.9	175	200	257	178	211	260	151	170	202	147	167	198
10–10.9	181	210	274	174	209	265	156	180	221	148	170	197
11–11.9	186	223	280	185	224	303	159	183	230	150	181	223
12–12.9	193	232	303	194	237	294	167	195	241	162	191	220
13–13.9	194	247	301	202	243	338	172	211	245	169	198	240
14–14.9	220	253	322	214	252	322	189	223	264	174	201	247
15–15.9	222	264	320	208	254	322	199	237	252	175	202	244
16–16.9	244	278	343	218	258	334	213	249	296	170	202	249
17–17.9	246	285	347	220	264	350	224	258	312	175	205	257
18–18.9	245	297	379	222	258	325	226	264	324	174	202	245
19–24.9	262	308	372	221	265	345	238	273	321	179	207	249
25–34.9	271	319	375	233	277	368	243	279	326	183	212	264
35–44.9	278	326	374	241	290	378	247	286	327	186	218	272
45–54.9	267	322	376	242	299	384	239	281	326	187	220	274
55–64.9	258	317	369	243	303	385	236	278	320	187	225	280
65–74.9	248	307	355	240	299	373	223	268	306	185	225	279

*Adapted from Frisancho AR. New norms of upper limb fat and muscle areas for assessment of nutritional status. *Am J Clin Nutr.* 1981, 343–2540

†The Lange caliper was used in these studies.

Table 4.
Normal Values for Maximal Inspiratory and Expiratory Respiratory Pressures for Adults

	Maximal Inspiratory Pressure (cm H_2O)		Maximal Expiratory Pressure (cm H_2O)	
Age Range (yr)	Male	Female	Male	Female
20–54	124±22	87±16	233±42	152±27
55–59	103±16	77±13	218±37	145±20
60–64	103±16	73±13	209±37	140±20
65–69	103±16	70±13	197±37	135±20
70–74	103±16	65±13	185±37	128±20

Values represent mean ±SD.
Adapted from Black LF, Hyatt RE. Maximal respiratory pressures: Normal values and relationship to age and sex. Am Rev Resp Dis 1969, 696.

Table 5.
Lower Limits of Acceptable Grip Strength Preoperatively*

Age	Female Grip Strength (kg)	Male Grip Strength (kg)
15	28	42
20	29	43
25	30	44
30	30	45
35	30	45
40	30	45
45	30	45
50	29	45
55	28	44
60	27	43
65	25	41
70	23	39
75	20	37
80	18	35
85	15	32
90	11	29
95	8	26

*85% Age-sex standard.
Webb AR, Newman LA, Taylor M, Keosh JB. Hands rip dynamometry as a predictor of postoperative complications. Reappraisal using age standardized grip strengths. JPEN 1989, 13:30–3.

Table 6.
Triceps Skinfold Thickness

Age (yr)	Males n	5	10	25	50	75	90	95	Females n	5	10	25	50	75	90	95
1–1.9	228	6	7	8	10	12	14	16	204	6	7	8	10	12	14	16
2–2.9	223	6	7	8	10	12	14	15	208	6	8	9	10	12	15	16
3–3.9	220	6	7	8	10	11	14	15	208	7	8	9	11	12	14	15
4–4.9	230	6	6	8	9	11	12	14	208	7	8	8	10	12	14	16
5–5.9	214	6	6	8	9	11	14	15	219	6	7	8	10	12	15	18
6–6.9	117	5	6	7	8	10	13	16	118	6	6	8	10	12	14	16
7–7.9	122	5	6	7	9	12	15	17	126	6	7	9	11	13	16	18
8–8.9	117	5	6	7	8	10	13	16	118	6	8	9	12	15	18	24
9–9.9	121	6	6	7	10	13	17	18	125	8	8	10	13	16	20	22
10–10.9	146	6	6	8	10	14	18	21	152	7	8	10	12	17	23	27
11–11.9	122	6	6	8	11	16	20	24	117	7	8	10	13	18	24	28
12–12.9	153	6	6	8	11	14	22	28	129	8	9	11	14	18	23	27
13–13.9	134	5	5	7	10	14	22	26	151	8	8	12	15	21	26	30
14–14.9	131	4	5	7	9	14	21	24	141	9	10	13	16	21	26	28
15–15.9	128	4	5	6	8	11	18	24	117	8	10	12	17	21	25	32
16–16.9	131	4	5	6	8	12	16	22	142	10	12	15	18	22	26	31
17–17.9	133	5	5	6	8	12	16	19	114	10	12	13	19	24	30	37
18–18.9	91	4	5	6	9	13	20	24	109	10	12	15	18	22	26	30
19–24.9	531	4	5	7	10	15	20	22	1,060	10	11	14	18	24	30	34
25–34.9	971	5	6	8	12	16	20	24	1,987	10	12	16	21	27	34	37
35–44.9	806	5	6	8	12	16	20	23	1,614	12	14	18	23	29	35	38
45–54.9	898	6	6	8	12	15	20	25	1,047	12	16	20	25	30	36	40
55–64.9	734	5	6	8	11	14	19	22	809	12	16	20	25	31	36	38
65–74.9	1503	4	6	8	11	15	19	22	1,670	12	14	18	24	29	34	36

Column header: Triceps Skinfold Percentiles (mm_2)*

*Percentiles for Triceps Skinfold for Whites of the United States Health and Nutrition Examination Survey 1 of 1971 to 1974

The Lange caliper was used in these studies.

Adapted from Frisancho AR. New norms of upper limb fat and muscle areas for assessment of nutritional status. Am J Clin Nutr 1981;34:2540.

Table 7.
Percentiles for Triceps Skinfold Thickness in the Elderly

Age Group (yr)	5%	50%	95%
Men			
65	8.6	13.8	27.0
70	7.7	12.9	26.1
75	6.8	12.0	25.2
80	6.0	11.2	24.3
85	5.1	10.3	23.4
90	4.2	9.4	22.6
Women			
65	13.5	21.6	33.0
70	12.5	20.6	32.0
75	11.5	19.6	31.0
80	10.5	18.6	30.0
85	9.5	17.6	29.0
90	8.5	16.6	28.0

Data are from 119 men and 150 women. All subjects are ambulatory, and measurements were made in the recumbent position on the left side. (Reprinted with permission from Chumlea WC, Roche AF, Mukherjee D. Nutritional Assessment for the Elderly Through Anthropometry. Ross Laboratories, Columbus, Ohio, 1984).

Table 8.
Lean Body Mass and Body Fat

	Male			Female		
Age*	LBM (kg)	Fat (kg)	%Fat	LBM (kg)	Fat (kg)	%Fat
Birth	3.06	0.49	14	2.83	0.49	15
6 mo	6.0	2.0	25	5.3	1.9	26
12 mo	7.9	2.3	22	7.0	2.2	24
2 yr	10.1	2.5	20	9.5	2.4	20
4 yr	14.0	2.7	16	13.2	2.8	18
6 yr	17.9	2.8	14	16.3	3.2	16
8 yr	22.0	3.3	13	20.5	4.3	17
10 yr	27.1	4.3	14	26.2	6.4	20
12 yr	34	8	19	32	10	24
14 yr	45	10	18	38	13	25
16 yr	57	9	14	42	13	24
18 yr	61	9	13	43	13	23
20 yr	62	9	13	43	14	25
22 yr	62	10	14	43	14	25

*At nearest birthday.

Table 9.
Non-protein Calorie to Nitrogen Ratio of Standard Parenteral Nutrition Solutions

Dextrose Concentration (%)	Dextrose Calories Per Liter (kcal)	Non-protein Calorie to Nitrogen Ratio for Amino Acid Concentration		
		2%	3.5%	4.25%
10	340	106	60	50
15	510	159	90	75
20	680	212	120	100
25	850	239	151	125
30	1020	318	181	150
35	1190	372	211*	175

*Not available as a standard solution.

Calories from parenteral fat emulsion must be included in calculating the final non-protein calorie to nitrogen ratio:

$$\frac{\text{Dextrose Calories + Fat Calories}}{\text{Amino Acids (g)}} \times 6.25 = \text{ratio}$$

Table 10.
Electrolyte Requirements

	Adult (Pediatric)
Sodium*	80 to 130 mEq/day (3–4 mEq/kg/day) as chloride, acetate salt or phosphate
Potassium	70 to 150 mEq/day (2–3 mEq/kg/day) as chloride, acetate or phosphate salt
Calcium	1.8 to 2.7 g/day (60–90 mg/kg/day or 90–135 mEq/day) as gluconate salt
Magnesium*	0.25 to 0.35 mEq/kg/day (0.25–0.5 mEq/kg/day) as sulfate salt
Phosphorous	930 to 1390 mg/day or 30–45 mmol/day (47–70 mg/kg/day)

*Increased with large losses present in gastrointestinal disease.

	Mineral Conversion Factors
Ca	20 mg = 1 mEq = 0.5 mmol
P	31 mg = 1 mmol
Na	23 mg = 1 mEq =1 mmol
K	39 mg = 1 mEq = 1 mmol
Mg	12 mg = 1 mEq = 0.5 mmol
Cl	35 mg = 1 mEq = 1 mmol

Table 11.
Food and Nutrition Board, National Academy for Sciences—National Research Council Recommended Daily Allowances (1989)

					Fat Soluble Vitamins			
	Age	Median Weight (kg)	Median Height (in)	Protein (g)	Vitamin A (mcg RE)	Vitamin D (mcg)	Vitamin E (mg Q-TE)	Vitmin K (mcg)
Infants	<6 mo	6	24	13	375	7.5	3	5
	6–12 mo	9	28	14	375	10	4	10
Children	1–3 yr	13	35	16	400	10	6	15
	4–6	20	44	24	500	10	7	20
	7–10	28	52	28	700	10	7	30
Males	11–14	45	62	45	1000	10	10	45
	15–18	66	69	59	1000	10	10	65
	19–24	72	70	58	1000	10	10	70
	25–50	79	70	63	1000	5	10	80
	>51	77	68	63	1000	5	10	80
Females	11–14	46	62	46	800	10	8	45
	15–18	55	64	44	800	10	8	55
	19–24	58	65	46	800	10	8	60
	25–50	63	64	50	800	5	8	65
	>51	65	63	50	800	5	8	65
Pregnant				60	800	10	10	65
Lactating	1st 6 mo			65	1300	10	12	65
	2nd 6 mo			62	1200	10	11	65

Table 12.
Food and Nutrition Board, National Academy for Sciences—National Research Council Recommended Daily Allowances (1989)

		Water-Soluble Vitamins						
	Age	Vitamin C (mg)	Vitamin B_1 (mg)	Riboflavin (mg)	Niacin (mg NE)*	Vitamin B_6 (mg)	Folate (mcg)	Vitamin B_{12} (mcg)
Infants	<6 mo	30	0.3	0.4	5	0.3	25	0.3
	6–12 mo	35	0.4	0.5	6	0.6	35	0.5
Children	1–3 yr	40	0.7	0.8	9	1.0	50	0.7
	4–6	45	0.9	1.1	12	1.1	75	1.0
	7–10	45	1.0	1.2	13	1.4	100	1.4
Males	15–18	60	1.5	1.8	20	2.0	200	2.0
	19–24	60	1.5	1.7	19	2.0	200	2.0
	25–50	60	1.5	1.7	19	2.0	200	2.0
	>51	60	1.2	1.4	15	2.0	200	2.0
Females	15–18	60	1.1	1.3	15	1.5	180	2.0
	19–24	60	1.1	1.3	15	1.6	180	2.0
	25–50	60	1.1	1.3	15	1.6	180	2.0
	>51	60	1.0	1.2	13	1.6	180	2.0
Pregnant		70	1.5	1.6	17	2.2	400	2.2
Lactating	1st 6 mo	95	1.6	1.8	20	2.1	280	2.6
	2nd 6 mo	90	1.6	1.7	20	2.1	260	2.6

*NE (niacin equivalent) = 1 mg niacin or 60 mg dietary tryptophan.

Table 13.
Food and Nutrition Board, National Academy for Sciences—National Research Council Recommended Daily Allowances (1989)

		Minerals						
	Age	Ca (mg)	P* (mg)	Mg (mg)	Fe (mg)	Zn (mg)	I (mcg)	Se (mcg)
Infants	<6 m	400	300	40	6	5	40	10
	6–12 mo	600	500	60	10	5	50	15
Children	1–3 yr	800	800	80	10	10	70	20
	4–6	800	800	120	10	10	90	20
	7–10	800	800	170	10	10	120	30
Males	15–18	1200	1200	400	12	15	150	50
	19–24	1200	1200	350	10	15	150	70
	25–50	800	800	350	10	15	150	70
	>51	800	800	350	10	15	150	70
Females	15–18	1200	1200	300	15	12	150	50
	19–24	1200	1200	280	15	12	150	55
	25–50	800	800	280	15	12	150	55
	>51	800	800	280	10	12	150	55
Pregnant		1200	1200	320	30	15	175	65
Lactating	1st 6 mo	1200	1200	355	15	19	200	75
	2nd 6 mo	1200	1200	340	15	16	200	75

*31 mg phosphorous is contained in 1 mmol phosphate.

Table 14.
Approximate Electrolyte Concentration of Body Fluids (mEq/L)

Source	Adult Volume Per Day	Na	K	Cl	HCO_3
Gastric	2000* to	60	20	90	—
	2500† ml	100	10	100	—
Pancreas	1000 ml	140	5	75	90
Bile	1500 ml	140	5	100	35
Small Bowel	3500 ml	140	15	100	25
Diarrhea	1000 to 4000 ml	60	30	45	45
Sweat	500 to 4000 ml	40–80	4	40–80	

*pH less than 4.
†pH greater than 4.

Table 15.
Electrolyte Abnormalities Associated with Parenteral Nutrition

Abnormality	Manifestations	Usual Causes
Hyponatremia	Weakness, confusion, seizures, lethargy, CHF	Na depletion, SIADH, renal failure
Hypernatremia	Weakness, confusion	Inadequate free lethargy, thirst H_2O in take
Hypokalemia	Weakness, cramps, cardiac ectopy	Inadequate intake, anabolic state
Hyperkalemia	Weakness, paresthesias cardiac arrhythmias	Excess intake, renal failure, acidosis
Hypocalcemia	Tetany, seizures, osteomalacia	Inadequate intake, sepsis, renal failure
Hypercalcemia	Lethargy, confusion	Excess intake, polyuria
Hypophosphatemia	Weakness, confusion, CNS changes, decreased WBC function	Inadequate intake, anabolic state
Hyperphosphatemia	Hypocalcemia, metastatic calcification	Excess intake, renal failure, acidosis
Hypomagnesemia	Hypocalcemia, renal potassium wasting	Inadequate intake, diuretics

Table 16.
Signs and Symptoms of Trace Element Deficiencies

Trace Element	Signs and Symptoms
Zinc	Anorexia, growth depression, dermatitis, hypogeusia, alopecia, impaired wound healing, immune suppression, night blindness, hypogonadism
Copper	Anemia (microcytic) leukopenia, neutropenia, osteoporosis, hair and skin depigmentation, poor connective tissue, neuropathy
Manganese	Growth depression, bone deformities, B-cell degeneration, retarded growth of hair and nails, transient dermatitis in animals
Chromium	Impaired glucose tolerance (?), elevated serum lipids (?), peripheral neuropathy
Iron	Anemia (microcytic)
Molybdenum	Growth retardation, impaired methionine and uric acid metabolism in animals
Iodine	Thyroid disease (goiter, hypothyroidism, cretinism)
Selenium	Cardiomyopathy, pseudoalbinism, macrocytic anemia, myositis, growth retardation, (?) cancer, infection
Silicon	Impaired growth, skeletal deformities, and connective tissue formation in animals
Fluoride	Caries, osteoporosis (?)
Cobalt	Pernicious anemia
Nickel	Growth retardation, impaired lipid metabolism in animals
Vanadium	Growth depression, impaired reproduction and lipid metabolism in animals

Table 17.
Classical Vitamin Deficiency States

Vitamins	Role	Deficiency State
Water-soluble		
Thiamine (B_1)	Co-enzyme in oxidative decarboxylation reactions	Beriberi: Cardiomyopathy Peripheral Neuropathy Encephalopathy
Riboflavin (B_2)	Co-enzyme of flavoproteins (FMN and FAD) involved in electron transport, tissue oxidation	Angular Stomatitis Glossitis Cheilosis Photophobia, tearing Seborrheic dermatitis (nasolabial fold and scrotum) Hypochromic anemia
Pantothenic acid	Precursor of Co-enzyme A involved in synthesis and fatty acids and steroid hormones	"Burning feet" syndrome Fatigue, leg cramps, paresthesias
Niacin	Constituent of the co-enzymes	Pellagra: (dementia, diarrhea, dermatitis)
	NAD and NADP involved in hydrogen transport, glycolysis	Scarlet, raw tongue Fissures of tongue
Pyridoxine (B_6)	Co-enzyme involved in amino acid metabolism and DNA synthesis	Peripheral neuropathy Convulsions Glossitis Cheilosis Seborrheic dermatitis (eyes, nose and mouth areas) Hypochromic anemia
Biotin	Co-enzyme in carboxylation reactions	Dermatitis Alopecia Depression Muscle pain Paresthesias
Folic acid	Co-enzyme in amino acid metabolism and DNA synthesis	Anemia (macrocytic) Stomatitis Diarrhea
B_{12}	Co-enzyme in amino acid metabolism and DNA synthesis	Anemia (megaloblastic) Neuropathy and paresthesias Glossitis
C	Connective tissue formation	Scurvy (weakness, irritability, bleeding gums, arthralgias, loosening of teeth)
	Oxidation/reduction reactions	Delayed wound healing Petechiae

Table 17. (*continued*)
Classical Vitamin Deficiency States

Vitamins	Role	Deficiency State
Fat-soluble vitamins		
A	Retinal pigment formation Epithelial integrity	Xerophthalmia Keratomalacia Night blindness Delayed wound healing Sterility (males)
D	Calcium and phosphate homeostasis	Rickets Osteomalacia
E	Antioxidant	Neuropathy (paresis of gaze, gait disturbance, decreased proprioception)
K	Synthesis of prothrombin factors II, VII, IX, X	Hemorrhage

Table 18.
Long-Term Central Venous Catheter and Care Chart (Adapted from UCLA Policies and Procedures)

Catheter Type	Description	Placement/Duration	Dressing Care/Hub Care	Heparin Flush	Clamps	Priming Volume	Special Considerations
PICC (Peripherally Inserted Central Catheter)	Silastic, silicone Elastomer CVC inserted peripherally via basilic or antecutibal vein into central circulation	• By RN, or MD at bedside • May stay in place up to 12 months or more	• Steri-strips, gauze and sterile transparent dressing q. week	150 units (100 U/ml) heparin per lumen q.d. when capped after meds, IVs	Use slide clamp on microbore extension set	0.6 ml	• Change microbore extension set q.4–6 weeks using sterile gloves • Never power push solution through catheter, may cause rupture • May develop post insertion phlebitis for 24–48h during first week after insertion. Treat with moist heat, rest, elevation of extremity. • 90% resolve without catheter removal
Tunneled CVCs **Single Lumen:** Broviac Hickman **Double Lumen:** Hickman, Quinton, RAAF	Tunneled silastic CVC with Dacron cuff designed for long-term access (also known as right atrial catheter)	• By MD in OR or surgical procedure area • May stay in place indefinitely	• Gauze and tape q.24–48hr, sterile transparent 1.3 × /wk • 3 × 3 HUB care • 30 second povidone-iodine prep on ports	300 U (100 U/ml) heparin per lumen q.d. when capped or after meds, IVs	Use preattached clamps on CVC or smooth jawed green plastic clamps	0.3–1.8 ml	• Appearance of Dacron cuff at exit site indicates dislodgement of line

Table 18. (*continued*)
Long-Term Central Venous Catheter and Care Chart (Adapted from UCLA Policies and Procedures)

Catheter Type	Description	Placement/Duration	Dressing Care/Hub Care	Heparin Flush	Clamps	Priming Volume	Special Considerations
Groshong Single or double lumen	Same as tunneled CVC but with slit valve at end of line to prevent reflux of blood into catheter	• By MD in OR or surgical procedure area • May stay in place indefinitely.	• Gauze and tape q.24–48hr, sterile transparent 1–3 × /wk • 3 × 3 HUB care • 30 second povidone-iodine prep on ports	• No heparin flush with 5 ml NS q.7 days when capped or after IV meds, fluids • Flush with 10 ml NS after blood draw • Flush with 20 ml NS prior to blood draw when TPN on	No clamps necessary because of slit valve	0.4–1.2 ml	• Line has blue and white stripes on silastic, yellow and red adapters on ends. Does not require heparin flush. Cannot be used to draw blood

Subcutaneous Infusion Port	Small metal chamber with self-sealing silicone rubber septum attached to silastic catheter implanted subcutaneously, accessed through skin via Huber needle	• By MD in OR or surgical procedure area • May stay in place indefinitely	• Sterile transparent dressing q.1–3 × /wk • 3 × 3 HUB care • 30 second povidone-iodine prep on ports	500 units U/ml) with 5 ml NS q. month when not in use or after IV meds, fluids	When needle in heparin (100 clamp on microbore extension set	1.2–2.1 ml place, use slide	• Change Huber needle q.week. • Confirm Huber needle placement prior to port use by aspiration of blood from port • Watch for bubbling leakage of fluid around port when flushing • Rotate site of needle to prevent fistula tract formation to port
Short-Term: (Peripherally Inserted Central Catheter) Single Lumen Double Lumen Triple Lumen Quadruple Lumen (EX: Arrowcath, Quadcath)	Single or multi-lumen catheter made of stiff plastic such as polyurethane or vinylchloride, placed percutaneously for short-term access up to 3 weeks	• By M.D. at bedside • May stay in place approximately 7–21 days	• Gauze and tape q.24h, sterile transparent q.M.W.F.	300 units (100 U/ml) heparin per lumen q.d. when capped, after IV meds, fluids	Use slide clamp on CVC or extension set	0.3–0.6 ml	Recommended lumen usage: distal: CVP readings, blood products, general access, medical: TPN, IV fluids, proximal: general access, venous blood draws

Table 19.
Osmolalities of Parenteral Nutrients

Nutrient	Concentration	mOsm/kg
Dextrose	10%	505
	20%	1010
	30%	1515
	40%	2020
	50%	2525
	60%	3030
	70%	3535
Fat emulsion	10%	276–300
	20%	258–350
Amino acids	8.5%	810
	10%	1000
Sodium chloride	4 mEq/mL	4.99
Sodium acetate	2 mEq/mL	4.0
Potassium chloride	2 mEq/mL	4.0
Potassium acetate	2 mEq/mL	4.0
Calcium chloride	1.36 mEq/mL	2.15
Calcium gluconate	0.46 mEq/mL	0.295

Table 20.
Calorie and Protein Chart for Selected Rates and Dextrose/Amino Acid Concentrations

Rate	Volume	Calories (kcal/day) Dextrose Concentrations		Protein (g/day) Amino Acid Concentration		
(ml/hr)	(ml/day)	10%	25%	2%	3.5%	4.25%
42	1000	340	850	20.0	35.0	42.5
50	1200	408	1020	24.0	42.0	51.0
60	1440	490	1224	28.8	50.4	61.2
70	1680	571	1428	33.6	58.8	71.4
80	1920	653	1632	38.4	67.2	81.6
83	2000	680	1700	40.0	70.0	85.0
90	2160	734	1836	43.2	75.6	91.8
100	2400	816	2040	48.0	84.0	102.0
110	2640	898	2244	52.8	92.4	112.2
120	2880	979	2448	57.6	100.8	122.4
125	3000	1020	2550	60.0	105.0	127.5

Table 21.
Energy Content of Parenteral Nutrients (kcal/ml)

Nutrient	% w/v (g/100 ml)	kcal/ml
Dextrose monohydrate	7.5	0.26
(3.4 kcal/g)	10.0	0.34
	12.0	0.41
	12.5	0.425
	15.0	0.51
	17.5	0.595
	20.0	0.68
	25.0	0.85
	30.0	1.00
	40.0	1.38
Protein (4 kcal/g)	1.0	0.04
	2.2	0.09
	2.3	0.092
	2.5	0.10
	2.7	0.11
	3.0	0.12
	4.0	1.16
Fat	10.0	1.10
	20.0	2.00

Examples of parenteral nutrition solutions:
1. Dextrose 12%; amino Acids 2.2%: 0.41 kcal/ml + 0.09 kcal/ml – 0.5 kcal/ml.
2. Dextrose 20%; amino Acids 3%: 0.58 kcal/ml + 0.12 kcal/ml – 0.8 kcal/ml.

Table 22.
Amino Acid Profiles of Standard Crystalline Amino Acid Solutions for Parenteral Use[*]

Amino acid	Travasol 10%	FreAmine III[†] 10%	Aminosyn[†] 15%	Novamine[†] 15%
Essential amino acids (g/dL)				
Lysine	0.58	0.73	1.58	1.18
Tryptophan	0.18	0.15	0.30	0.25
Phenylalanine	0.56	0.56	0.45	1.04
Methionine	0.40	0.53	0.26	0.75
Threonine	0.42	0.40	0.60	0.75
Leucine	0.73	0.91	1.50	1.04
Isoleucine	0.60	0.69	0.99	0.75
Valine	0.58	0.66	0.75	0.96
Non-essential amino acids (g/dL)	0.48	0.28	0.45	0.89
Histidine	—	—	—	0.57
Glutamate	0.68	1.12	1.08	0.89
Proline	—	—	—	0.33
Aspartate	0.50	0.59	0.80	0.59
Serine	1.15	0.95	1.53	1.47
Arginine	2.07	0.71	1.49	2.17
Alanine	1.03	1.40	0.75	1.04
Glycine	0.04	—	0.40	0.39
Tyrosine	—	<0.02	1.05	0.43
Cysteine			1.11	0.75
Glutamic acid				

[*]Values given for the most single concentrated solution available in each product line.
[†]Contains sodium bisulfite as a preservative.
Aminosyn and Novamine data extrapolated to 10% solution equivalent.

Table 23.
Amino Acid Profiles of Modified Crystalline Amino Acid Solutions for Specialized Parenteral Use*

	Increased Essential Amino Acids				Increased Branch-Chain Amino Acids				Neonatal Formula
Amino Acid	Aminess® 5.2%	Aminosyn®© RF 5.2%	Nephramine II®© 5.4%	RenAmin® 6.5%	Aminosyn®© HBC 7%	Branchamin® 4%	FreAmine®© HBC 6.9%	HepatAmine®© 8%	Trophamine®© 6%
Essential amino acids (g/dL)	0.60	0.54	0.64	0.45	0.25	—	0.41	0.61	0.49
Lysine	0.19	0.16	0.20	0.16	0.09	—	0.09	0.07	0.12
Tryptophan	0.82	0.73	0.88	0.49	0.23	—	0.32	0.10	0.29
Phenylalanine	0.82	0.73	0.88	0.50	0.21	—	0.25	0.10	0.20
Methionine	0.38	0.33	0.40	0.38	0.27	—	0.20	0.45	0.25
Threonine	0.82	0.73	0.88	0.60	1.58	1.38	1.37	1.10	0.84
Leucine	0.52	0.46	0.56	0.50	0.79	1.38	0.76	0.90	0.49
Isoleucine	0.60	0.53	0.64	0.82	0.79	1.24	0.88	0.84	0.47
Valine									
Non-essential amino acids (g/dL)									
Histidine†	0.41	0.43	0.25	0.42	0.15	—	0.16	0.24	0.29
Glutamate	—	—	—	—	—	—	—	—	0
Proline	—	—	—	0.35	0.45	—	0.63	0.80	0.41
Aspartate	—	—	—	—	—	—	—	—	0
Serine	—	—	—	0.30	0.22	—	0.33	0.50	0.23
Arginine	—	0.60	—	0.63	0.51	—	0.58	—	0.73
Alanine	—	—	—	0.56	0.66	—	0.40	0.77	0.32
Glycine	—	—	—	0.30	0.66	—	0.33	0.90	0.22
Tyrosine	—	—	—	0.04	0.03	—	—	—	0.14
Cysteine	—	—	<0.02	—	—	—	<0.02	<0.02	<0.02
Taurine	—	—	—	—	—	—	—	—	0.015

*Value given for a single concentrated solution available in each product line.
†Histidine is considered essential for patients with renal failure.
Contains sodium bisulfite.

Table 24.
Average Daily Calories from Parenteral Fat Emulsion Dosing Regimens

Dosing	10% Fat		20% Fat			
Frequency	100 ml	500 ml	100 ml	200 ml	250 ml	500 ml
Q D	110	550	200	400	500	1000
Q O D	55	275	100	200	250	500
Q 3 D	37	183	67	114	167	333
1 day/wk	16	79	29	57	71	143
2 day/wk	31	157	57	114	143	286
3 day/wk	47	236	86	171	214	429
4 day/wk	63	314	114	229	286	571
5 day/wk	79	393	143	286	357	714
6 day/wk	94	471	171	343	429	857

Table 25.
Comparison of Two Commercially Available Intravenous Lipid Emulsions

	Intralipid®	Liposyn II®
Composition (g/100 mL, %)		
Egg yolk phospholipids	1.2	1.2
Glycerol	2.5	2.5
Soybean oil	10	10
Fatty acid content (%)		
Linoleic acid	54	54.5
Linolenic acid	8	8.3
Oleic acid	26	22.4
Palmitic acid	9	10.5
Stearic acid	2.5	4.2
Osmolality (mOsm)	280	300
Caloric density (kcal/mL)	1.1	1.1
Vitamin E and PUFA content		
Alpha-tocopherol (mg/dL)	<1	20.0
Gamma-tocopherol (mg/dL)	12.0	0
Vitamin E activity (mg/L)	1.4	20.0
(units/L)	2.1	29.8
PUFA (g/L)	62.0	77.0
Vitamin E: PUFA ratio	0.02	0.26

PUFA = polyunsaturated fatty acid.

Table 26.
Composition of Parenteral Multiple Vitamin Formulations

Vitamin	Multi-Vitamins for Infusion* (10 ml)	Key-Plex® Vitamin B Complex Plus C (1 ml)	MVI Pediatric® 5ml†
Vitamin A (RE)	3300	0	2300
Vitamin D (IU)	200	0	400
Vitamin E (IU)	10	0	7
Thiamine (mg)	3	50	1.2
Riboflavin (mg)	3.6	5	1.4
Niacinamide (mg)	40	125	17
Pyridoxine (mg)	4	5	1
Dexpanthenol (mg)	15	6	5
Vitamin C (mg)	100	50	805.0
Folic Acid (mcg)	400	0	140
Vitamin B_{12} (mcg)	5	1000	1
Vitamin K (mg)	0	0	0.2
Biotin (mcg)	60	0	20

*These quantities are identical to the guidelines of the American Medical Association, Nutrition Advisory Group for parenteral multivitamins in adults (1979).
†Use 2 ml/kg body wt. for infants. Max. dose is 5 ml per day.

Table 27.
Recommended Daily Intravenous Intake of Essential Trace Elements

	Stable Adult	Acute Adult Catabolic State*	Stable Adult with Intestinal Losses*
Zinc	2.5–4.0 mg	Additional 2.0 mg 400 g/kg	Add 12.2 mg/l small bowel fluid lost; 17.1 mg/l of stool or ileostomy output
Iodine	?	1.0 μg/kg/day	—
Copper	0.5–1.5 mg	−20 μg/kg	—
Chromium†	10–15 mcg	−0.2 μg/kg	
Manganese†	0.15–0.8 mg	−1 μg/kg	—
Selenium‡	40–120 mcg	?	—

	Pre-Term Infant	Term Infant	Children
Zinc	400 mcg/kg/day	250 mcg/kg/day <3 m 100 mcg/kg/day >3 m	50 mcg/kg/d max. 5000 mcg/day
Copper	20 mcg/kg/day	20 mcg/kg/day	20 mcg/kg/day max. 300 mcg/day
Chromium	0.20 mcg/kg/day	0.20 mcg/kg/day	0.20 mcg/kg/day max. 5.0 mcg/day
Magnesium	1.0 mcg/kg/day	1.0 mcg/kg/day	2.0 mcg/kg/day max. 50 mcg/day
Selenium‡	2.0 mcg/kg/day	2.0 mcg/kg/day	2.0 mcg/kg/day max. 30 mcg/day

Frequent monitoring of blood concentrations in these patients is essential to provide proper dosage.
*American Medical Association, Department of Food & Nutrition. Guidelines for Essential Trace Element Preparations for Parenteral Use. JAMA 1979; 241(19):2051–2054, Amer J Clin Nutr 48:1324–33, 1988.
†Deficiency state in humans not conclusively identified
‡Not described by the AMA

Table 28.
Medications That Can Be Co-infused with IV Fat Emulsions

Cefamandole sodium	Cefazolin sodium
Cefoxitin sodium	Clindamycin
Digoxin	Dopamine HCl
Erythromycin	Furosemide
Gentamycin	Heparin
Hydrocortisone sodium succinate	Isoproterenol HCl
Insulin (regular)	Lidocaine HCl
Methyldopate HCl (in NS)	Methylprednisolone sodium succinate
Metoclopramide	Norepinephrine HCl
Oxacillin sodium	Penicillin G sodium or potassium
Ticarcillin	Tobramycin

Table 29.
Medications That May Be Piggybacked into Amino Acid/Dextrose Solution

Albumin	Amikacin sulfate
Aminophylline	Azlocillin sodium
Aztreonam	Carbenicillin disodium
Cefamandole sodium	Cefazolin sodium
Cefoperazone sodium	Cefoxitin
Cefotaxime sodium	Ceftriaxone sodium
Ceftazidime	Cefuroxime
Cephalothin sodium	Cephapirin sodium
Cephradine	Cimetidine
Chloramphenicol	Clindamycin
Cyclophosphamide	Cytarabine
Digoxin	Dobutamine
Dopamine HCl	Doxycycline
Erythromycin	5-Fluorouracil
Furosemide	Gentamicin
Heparin	Hydrocortisone sodium succinate
Hydromorphone HCl	Imipenem
Insulin (regular)	Isoproterenol HCl
Levarterenol bitartrate	Leucovorin calcium
Lidocaine HCl	Meperidine HCl
Metaraminol bitartrate	Methicillin sodium
Methotrexate sodium	Methyldopate HCI (in NS)
Methylprednisolone sodium succinate	Metoclopramide HCl
Mezlocillin	Miconazole
Morphine sulfate	Moxalactam sodium
Nafcillin sodium	Norepinephrine
Oxacillin sodium	Penicillin G sodium or potassium
Piperacillin	Ranitidine
Tetracycline	Ticarcillin
Tobramycin	Urokinase
Vancomycin	

Table 30.
Normal Nutritional Values in Children

Test	Normal Value	Exceptions
Protein		
Blood		
Serum albumin (g/dL)	≥3.5	≥2.5–3 for Infant
Retinal binding protein (mg/dL)	3–6	2–3 children <9 yr
Blood urea nitrogen (mg/dL)	7–22	
Thyroxin binding protein (mg/dL)	20–50	
Transferrin (mg/dL)	170–250	
Fibronectin (mg/dL)	30–40	
Urine		
Creatinine/height index	>0.9	
3-methyl histidine (uMol/kg)	3.2 ± 0.6 male 2.1 ± 0.4 female 4.2 ± 1.3 neonate	
3-methyl histidine (uMol/gm creatinine)	126 ± 32 male 92 ± 23 female 253 ± 78 neonate	
Hydroxyproline index	>2	
Vitamin A		
Plasma retinol (mg/dL)	≥30	
Plasma retinol binding protein (mg/dL)	2–3	
Vitamin D		
25-OH-D_3 (ng/ml)	≥20	
Riboflavin		
Red cell gluthatione reductase simulation (%)	<20	
Vitamin B_6		
Red cell transaminases Plasma pyridoxal phosphate Xanthurenic acid excretion	Feasible and useful in all age groups but not readily available and not practical in children <9 years of age	
Folacin		
Serum folate (ng/ml)	>6	
Red blood cell folate (ng/ml)	>160	
Vitamin K		
Prothrombin time (seconds)	11–15	
Vitamin E		
Plasma alpha-tocopherol (mg/dL)	≥0.7	
Red blood hemolysis test (%)	≤10	
Vitamin C		
Plasma (mg/dL)	>0.2	
Leukocyte (mg/100 cells)	Difficult to perform on children due to sample requirements	

Table 30. (*continued*)
Normal Nutritional Values in Children

Test	Normal Value	Exceptions
Thiamine		
Red blood cell transketolase stimulation (%)	<15	
Vitamin B_{12}		
Serum vitamin B_{12} (pg/ml)	≥200	
Absorption test	Excretion of more than 7.5% of ingested labeled Vitamin B_{12}	
Phosphorus	5–8 mg/dl	
Iron		
Hematocrit (%)	39	31 for neonate 33 for infant 36 for child and menstruating females
Hemoglobin (g/dL)	14	11 for neonate 12 for infant 13 for child and menstruating females
Serum ferratin (ng/ml)	>10	
Serum iron (ug/dL)	>60	>30 for neonate >40 for infant >50 for child <4 yr
Serum total iron binding Capacity (ug/dL)	350–400	
Serum transferrin saturation (%)	>16	>12 for infant >14–15 for child <9 yr
Serum transferrin (mg/dL)	170–250	
Erythrocyte protoporphyrin (ug/dL rbcs)	<70	<80 neonate <75 infant
Zinc		
Serum zinc (ug/dL)	60–120	
Erythrocyte zinc	Erythrocytes contain approximately 10 times more zinc than plasma	

Table 31.
Peripheral Parenteral Nutrition Solutions for Children

Neonate/Infant		Child (1–10 yr)	
Dextrose	12.5 gm	Dextrose	12.5 gm
Amino acids	2.2 gm	Amino acids	2.2 gm
NaCl (2.6 mEq)	2.6 mmol	NaCl (2.6 mEq)	2.6 mmol
KH_2PO_4-K_2HPO_4 (2.8 mmol K)	1.5 mmol P	KH_2PO_4-K_2HPO_4 (0.9 mmol K)	0.6 mmol P
Ca gluconate (48 mg Ca)	1.2 mmol	Ca gluconate (20 mg Ca)	0.5 mmol
$MgSO_4$ (6 mg Mg)	0.5 mEq	$MgSO_4$ (9.6 mg Mg)	0.8 mEq
KCI (0.2 mmol)	0.2 mmol	KCl (0.8 mmol)	0.8 mEq
Total K = 3.0 mEq or mmol		Total K = 1.7 mEq or Mmol	
Adolescent			
Dextrose	12.5 gm		
Amino acids	2.2 gm		
NaCl (4 mEq)	4.0 mmol		
KH_2PO_4-K_2HPO_4 (0.7 mEq K)	0.5 mmol P		
Ca gluconate (20 mg Ca)	0.5 mmol		
$MgSO_4$ (12 mg Mg)	1.0 mEq		
KCl (2 mmol)	2.0 mEq		
Total K = 2.7 mEq or mmol			

(0.5 kcal/ml): Components per dl (100 mL).

Table 32.
Central Parenteral Nutrition Solutions for Children

Nenoate/Infant (0.5 kcal/ml)		Child (1–10 yr) (0.8 kcal/ml)	
Dextrose	12.5 gm	Dextrose	20.0 gm
Amino Acids	2.2 gm	Amino Acids	3.0 gm
NaCl (2.6 mEq)	2.6 mmol	NaCl (3.8 mEq)	3.8 mmol
KH_2PO_4-K_2HPO_4 (1.8 mmol K)	1.2 mmol P	KH_2PO_4-K_2HPO_4 (1.5 mmol K)	1.0 mmol P
Ca gluconate (48 mg Ca)	1.2 mEq	Ca gluconate (36 mg Ca)	0.9 mmol
$MgSO_4$ (6 mg Mg)	0.5 mmol	$MgSO_4$ (9.6 mg Mg)	0.8 mEq
KCl	0.2 mEq	KCl (1.3 mEq)	1.3 mEq
Total K = 2.4 mEq or mmol		Total K = 2.8 mEq or mmol	
Adolescent (0.8 kcal/mL)			
Dextrose	20.0 gm		
Amino Acids	3.0 gm		
NaCl (6 mEq)	6.0 mmol		
KH_2PO_4-K_2HPO_4 (0.7 mmol K)	0.5 mmol P		
Ca gluconate (20 mg Ca)	0.5 mmol		
$MgSO_4$ (12 mg Mg)	1.0 mEq		
KCl (3 mEq)	3.0 mmol		
Total K = 3.7 mEq or 3.7 mmol			

Components per dl (100 ml).

Table 33.
Recommended Admixtures for Children

Solution 1 (1.0 kcal/mL)	
Dextrose	14.0 gm
Amino acids (Novamine® or Freamine III®)	3.0 gm
NaCl (6.2 meq)	6.2 mmol
KH_2PO_4-K_2HPO_4 (1.2 mmol K)	0.8 mmol P
Ca gluconate (16 mg Ca = 0.8 mEq)	0.4 mmol
$MgSO_4$ (9.6 mg Mg = 0.8 mEq)	0.4 mmol
KCl (3 mEq)	3.0 mmol
Trace minerals	Appropriate for age
Vitamins	Appropriate for age
Fat emulsion (Intralipid)	4.0 gm
Heparin	1 U/ml
Solution 2 (1.5 kcal/mL)	
Dextrose	25.0 gm
Amino acids (Novamine® or Freamine III®)	4.0 gm
NaCl (9.4 mEq)	9.4 mmol
KH_2PO_2-K_2HPO_4 (1.2 mEq K)	1.2 mmol P
Ca Gluconate (24 mg Ca)	0.6 mmol
$MgSO_4$ (14.4 mg Mg = 1.2 mEq)	0.6 mmol
KCl (3 mEq)	3.0 mmol
Trace minerals	Appropriate for age
Vitamins	Appropriate for age
Fat emulsion (Intralipid)	4.0 gm
Heparin	1 U/ml

Components per dl (100 ml).

Table 34.
Home TPN Solutions for Children (0.8 kcal/ml)

Infant		Child (1–10 yr)	
Dextrose	20.0 g	Dextrose	20.0 g
Amino acids	2.5 g	Amino acids	3.0 g
NaCl (2.6 mEq)	2.6 mEq	NaCl	3.8 mEq
KH_2PO_4-K_2HPO_4 (2.2 mmol K)	1.5 mmol	KH_2PO_4-K_2HPO_4 (1.5 mmol K)	1.0 mmol
Ca gluconate (40 mg Ca)	2.0 mEq	Ca gluconate (34 mg Ca)	1.7 mEq
$MgSO_4$ (9.6 mg Mg = 0.8 mEq)	0.8 mEq	$MgSO_4$ (9.6 mg Mg = 0.8 mEq)	0.8 mEq
KCl	0.2 mEq	KCl	1.3 mEq
Total K = 2.4 mEq or mmol		Total K = 2.8 mEq or mmol	
Trace Minerals	0.1 mL/kg/day	Trace Minerals	0.1 ml/kg/day
Vitamins (MVI®-Pediatric)	1 vial/day	Vitamins (MVI®-Pediatrics)	1 vial/day
Heparin	1 U/ml	Heparin	1 U/ml

Adolescent	
Dextrose	20.0 g
Amino Acids	3.0 g
NaCl	6.0 mEq
K_2HPO_4 (0.7 mEq K)	0.5 mmol
Ca gluconate (20 mg Ca)	1.0 mEq
$MgSO_4$ (6 mg Mg = 0.5 mEq)	0.5 mEq
KCl	3.0 mEq
Total K = 3.7 mEq or Mmol	
Trace Minerals (MTE 5)	4 ml/day
Vitamins (MVI® 12)	1 vial/day
Heparin	1 U/ml
Vitamin K 10.0 mg added 1 × /wk	

This home TPN solution is lower in Ca and P than the solution used in the hospital. The hospital solution cannot be used at home because during storage, calcium and phosphorus are likely to precipitate.
Fat emulsions will be required if TPN is supplying greater than 50% of caloric needs and/or food intake is not providing 4% of calories as essential fatty acids.
Components per dl (100 ml).

Table 35.
Composition of Milks

	g/100 ml			mg/100 ml			Source		Osmolality (mOsm/kg of H_2O) and General Comments
	Pro	Fat	CHO	Na K	Ca P	Fe	CHO	Fat	
Human milk (21 kcal/30 ml)	1.0	3.5	7.0	17 53	26 14	0.2	Lactose	Human Milk Fat	(280) Fe Supplementation recommended. Whey: casein ratio is 60:40 Page Lactation Consultant for questions
Whole cow's milk (18.8 kcal/30 ml)	3.3	3.3	4.6	51 146	120 95	TR	Lactose	Butterfat	(279) Not recommended for infants < 1 yr of age Whey:casein ratio is 18:82
2% milk (15.1 kcal/30 ml)	3.4	2.0	4.9	51 157	124 97	TR	Lactose	Butterfat	(279) Used to moderately reduce calories and fat. Not recommended for infants < 2 yr of age
Skim milk (10.8 kcal/30 ml)	3.5	0.2	5.0	53 169	126 103	TR	Lactose	Trace Butterfat	(279) Deficient in essential fatty acids. Not recommended for children < 2 yr of age
Evaporated whole milk (32 kcal/30 ml) (undiluted)	7.2	7.9	10.6	111 318	274 212	0.2	Lactose	Butterfat	Milk is diluted and sugar added to make a 20 calorie/oz formula
Goat's milk (21 kcal/30 ml)	3.6	4.2	4.5	51 208	136 112	TR	Lactose	Butterfat	(267) Casein more readily digested than casein in cow's milk

Table 36.
Standard Milk-Based Formulas for Infants

	gm/100m			mg/100 ml			Source		Osmolality (mOsm/kg of H_2O) and General Comments
	Pro	Fat	CHO	Na K	Ca P	Fe	CHO	Fat	
Similac® (Ross) (20 kcal/30 ml)	1.45	3.6	7.2	18 71	49 38 (w	0.15 iron	Lactose 1.2)	Coconut Oil Soy Oil	(300) Whey:Casein ratio is 18:82 Comments
Similac® (24 kcal/30 ml)	2.2	4.3	8.5	28 107	73 57 (w	0.18 iron	Lactose 1.5)	Coconut Oil Soy Oil	(380) Whey:Casein ratio is 18:82 Available for hospital use only.
Similar Concentrate® mixed to 24 kcal/oz	2.6	4.3	8.5	28 107	73 84	1.4	Lactose	Coconut Oil Soy Oil	Prepared from standard Similac concentrate, patient requires formula instruction prior to discharge
Similac® (27 kcal/30 ml)	2.5	4.8	9.5	31 121	82 64	1.4	Lactose	Coconut Oil Soy Oil	(410) Whey:Case.n ratio is 18:82

Enfamil® (Mead Johnson) (20 Kcal/30 ml)	1.5	3.8	6.9	18 72	52 35 (w	0.1 iron	Lactose 1.3)	Palm Olein Soy Oil Coconut Oil Sunflower Oil	(300) Whey:Casein ratio is 60:40
SMA® (Wyeth) (20 kcal/30 ml)	1.5	3.6	7.2	15 56	42 28	1.2	Lactose	Coconut Oil Safflower Oil, Oleo, Soy Oil	(300) Milk-based formula with low renal solute load. Whey:Casein ratio is 60:40
Gerber®	1.5	3.6	7.3	16 65	43 24	1.0	Lactose Malto- dextrins	Palm Oil Soy Oil Coconut Oil, Sunflower Oil	(320) Whey:Casein ratio is 18:82
Good Start®	1.6	3.4	7.3	16 65	43 24	1.0	Lactose Malto- dextrins	Palm Oil Oleic, Safflower Oil, Corn Oil	(260) Hydrolyzed Whey protein formula

Table 37.
Soy-Based Formulas for Infants

	gm/100m			mg/100 mL			Source		Osmolality (mOsm/kg of H_2O) and General Comments
	Pro	Fat	CHO	Na/K	Ca/P	Fe	CHO	Fat	
Isomil® (Ross) (20 kcal/30 ml)	1.8	3.7	6.8	30/73	71/51	1.2	Corn Syrup Solids; Sucrosa	Soy Oil, Coconut Oil	(240) Soy protein isolate formula. Lactose free formula
Isomil SF® (Ross) (20 kcal/30 ml)	1.8	3.7	6.8	30/73	71/51	1.2	Hydro-lyzed Corn starch	Soy Oil, Coconut Oil	(180) Soy protein isolate formula. Lactose and sucrose free.
Prosobee® (Mead Johnson) (20 kcal/30 ml)	2.0	3.5	6.7	24/81	63/49	1.3	Corn Syrup Solids	Palm Olein Coconut Oil, Soy Oil, Sunflower Oil	(200) Soy protein isolate formula. Lactose and sucrose free.
Nursoy® (Wyeth) (20 kcal/30ml)	1.8	3.6	6.9	20/70	60/42	1.2	Sucrose	Oleo, Coconut Oil, Safflower Oil, Soy Oil	(244) Soy protein isolate formula, Lactose free, no corn syrup solids.
I-Soylac® (Loma Linda) (20 kcal/30 ml)	2.1	3.7	6.7	28/78	68/47	1.3	Sucrose, Tapioca starch	Soy Oil	(206) Soy protein isolate formula. Corn free. Lactose free. Fe fortified.
Soyalac® (Loma Linda) (20 kcal/30 ml)	2.1	3.7	6.7	29/78	63/37	1.3	Corn Syrup Solids, Soy, Sucrose	Soy Oil	(273) Soy protein isolate formula. Lactose free. Fe fortified.

Table 38.
Specialized Infant Formulas

	g/100ml		mg/100ml				Source		Osmolality (mOsm/kg of H_2O) and General Comments
	Pro	Fat	CHO	Na	Ca	Fe	CHO	Fat	
Alimentum® (Ross) (20 kcal/30 ml)	1.9	3.8	6.8	29 79	70 50	1.2	Sucrose, Modified Tapioca Starch	MCT Oil, Safflower Oil, Soy Oil	(370) For malabsorption problems. Protein is casein hydrolysate with added amino acids. 50% fat from MCT oil.
Nutramigen® (Mead Johnson) (20 kcal/30ml)	1.9	2.6	8.9	31 73	63 42	1.3	Corn Syrup Solids, Modified Corn Starch	Corn Oil, Soy Oil	(320) For malabsorption problems. Protein is casein hydrolysate with added amino acids.
Pregestimil® (Mead Johnson) (20 kcal/30 ml)	1.9	3.7	6.9	26 73	62 42	1.3	Corn Syrup Solids, Modified Corn Starch, Dextrose	MCT Oil Corn Oil Soy Oil Safflower Oil	(300) For malabsorption problems. Protein is casein hydrolysate with added amino acids. 55% fat from MCT oil.
Pregestimil® (24 kcal/30 ml)	2.3	4.4	8.3	31 88	74 50	1.6	Same as Pregestimil 20	Same as Pregestimil 20	(360) For malabsorption problems. Patient needs formula instruction prior to discharge.
Portagen® (Mead Johnson) (20 kcal/ml)	2.3	3.2	7.7	37 83	63 47	1.3	Corn Syrup Solids, Sucrose	MCT Oil Corn Oil	(220) Medium chain triglyceride formula for LCT intolerance. Protein is sodium caseinate. 87% MCT oil.

Table 38. (*continued*)
Specialized Infant Formulas

	g/100ml		mg/100ml				Source		Osmolality (mOsm/kg of H_2O) and General Comments
	Pro	Fat	CHO	Na	Ca	Fe	CHO	Fat	
Lofenalac® (Mead Johnson) (20 kcal/30 ml)	2.2	2.6	8.7	31 68	83 83	1.3	Corn Syrup Solids, Modified Tapioca Starch	Corn Oil	(360) Low phenylalanine formula used in treatment of PKU. Protein is specially processed casein hydrolysate reduced in phenylalanine with other added amino acids.
Phenyl-Free® (Mead-Johnson) (20 kcal/30 ml)	3.3	1.1	10.7	66 223	55 37	1.9	Sucrose, Corn Syrup Solids, Modified Tapioca Starch	Corn Oil, Coconut Oil	Whey protein. Low calcium formula.
Lacto-Free® (Mead Johnson) (20 kcal/30ml)	1.5	3.6	6.9	20 73	38 19	1.1	Corn Syrup	Palm Oil, Soy Oil, Coconut Oil, Sunflower Oil	Protein provided as amino acids without phenylalanine.

Similac PM 60/40® (Ross) (20 kcal/30ml)	1.5	3.8	6.9	$\frac{16}{58}$	$\frac{16}{19}$	0.15	Lactose	Soy Oil, Coconut Oil	(200) For lactose intolerance, lactose free, mild protein isolate. Whey:Casein ratio is 20:80.
S-29 (Wyeth) (20 kcal/30ml)	1.7	2.2	9.8	$\frac{1.0}{32}$	$\frac{7}{18}$	1.3	Lactose	Oleo Coconut Oil Safflower Oil Soybean Oil	(280) Low renal solute load. Minerals comparable to human milk. Lactalbumin:Casein and Calcium:Phosphorus ratios comparable to human milk. Low iron formula.
Calcilo XD® (Wyeth) (20 kcal/30ml)	1.6	4.1	7.5	$\frac{16}{60}$		1.3	Lactose	Corn Oil, Coconut Oil	(360) Very low renal solute load. Whey protein.

Table 39.
Formulas Designed for Low Birth Weight Infants

	g/100 ml			mg/100 ml			Source		Osmolality (mOsm/kg of H_2O) and General Comments
	Pro	Fat	CHO	Na / K	Ca / P	Fe	CHO	Fat	
Enfamil Premature, Iron-Fortified® (Mead Johnson) 24 kcal/30 ml	2.4	4.0	8.8	31 / 82	131 / 66	1.5* (Low •Fe 0.2)	Corn Syrup Solids, Lactose	Soy Oil MCT Oil, Coconut Oil	(310) For low birth weight infants. Available for hospital use only. Whey:Casein ratio is 60:40. 40% fat from MCT oil.
Similac Special Care Iron-Fortified® (Ross) (24 kcal/30 ml)	2.2	4.4	8.6	35 / 105	146 / 73	1.5 (Low •Fe 0.3)	Lactose, Hydro-lyzed Corn Starch	MCT Oil Soy Oil, Coconut Oil	(280) For low birth weight infants. Available for hospital use only. Whey:Casein ratio 60:40. 50% fat from MCT oil. Recommended vitamin D supplement 400 IU/d.
Similac Special Care® (Ross) (20 kcal/30 ml)	1.8	3.6	7.1	29 / 87	122 / 61	0.2	Lactose, Hydro-lyzed Corn Starch	MCT Oil Soy Oil, Coconut Oil	(235) Available for hospital use only.

Similac Natural Care® (Ross) (24 kcal/30 ml)	2.2	4.4	8.6	35 104	170 85	—	Hydro- lyzed Corn- starch, Lactose	MCT Oil Soy Oil, Coconut Oil	Designed to be mixed with human milk or to be fed alternately with human milk to low birth weight infants.
Enfamil Human Milk Fortifier with EBM®† (Mead Johnson) @ 4 pk/100 ml	1.7	3.5	9.7	27 68.6	116 59	0.2	Glucose polymers, Lactose	—	(380) For low birth weight infants, or infants with volume restriction on expressed breast milk. Available for hospital use only. Whey:Casein ratio 60:40. Recommended mixture is 2 pk of fortifier/100 ml human milk for 24 hr, afterwards increased to 4 pk/100 ml human milk for 24 hr, afterwards increased to 4 pk/100 cc for full fortification. Does not contain iron.

*Also available as low iron formula.
†Expressed breast milk.

Table 40.
Modular Formulas for Infants

	g/100 ml			mg/100 ml			Source		Osmolality (mOsm/kg of H_2O) and General Comments
	Pro	Fat	CHO	Na / K	Ca / P	Fe	CHO	Fat	
RCF® (Ross) (12.1 kcal/30 ml at normal dilution with-out CHO)	2.0	3.6	0	30 / 73	70 / 50	0.15	none	Soy Oil Coconut Oil	(64 without added CHO) Used for those unable to tolerate the type or amount of carbohydrate in standard formulas. Should not be used without added carbohydrate.
Product 80056 (Mead Johnson) (17 kcal/30 ml with-out added protein and/or amino acids)	0	2.6	8.3 8.3	19 / 71	63 / 35	1.3	Corn Syrup, Modified Tapioca Starch	Corn Oil	Protein-free formula. For infants requiring specific mixtures of amino acids. Adequate protein or amino acids, sodium and potassium must be added.

Product 3232 A (Mead Johnson) (12.7 kcal/30 ml without added CHO)	1.9	2.8	2.8	29 73	63 42	1.3	Modified Tapioca Starch	MCT Oil Corn Oil	(250 without added CHO) Mono- and disaccharide-free powder for use with added carbohydrate. Used for disaccharidase deficiencies and for intractable diarrhea management. See Table 25F for adding CHO.
ProViMin® (Ross) (3.13 kcal/30 ml without added CHO or fat	2.2	0	0	35 97	71 50	1.1	none	none	A protein/mineral modular formula for use in special feedings for infants intolerant of usual amounts or types of carbohydrate and/or fat present in conventional feedings. Appropriate amounts of CHO, fat, essential vitamins and fatty acids must be added. See Table 25F.

Table 41.
Infant Carbohydrate-Protein-Fat Modula Additives

Ingredient	Calories	g/Tbsp	Source	Comments
Polycose Powder® Polycose Liquid® (Ross)	3.76/g 2/ml	6 15	Glucose Polymers	Carbohydrate which provides lower osmolality and minimal sweetness. Derived from corn starch.
Dextrose	3.8g	10	Corn Sugar	Anhydrous disaccharide used to increase calories.
Fructose	4/g	10	Fruit Sugar	Monosaccharide added to formula to increase calories for infants allergic to corn sugar or intolerant to other carbohydrates.
Sucrose	4/g	12	Cane or beet sugar	Disaccharide added to formula to increase calories.
Corn Syrup	2.9/g 3.8 ml	20	Corn Syrup	Added to increase calories. Contains corn syrup, sugar, vanilla and salt. 150 mg Na/100 g.
Casac® (Mead Johnson)	3.7g	4.7	Calcium Caseinate	Protein powder used to increase protein in formulas. 88% protein 1.6 % calcium. 150 mg Na/100 g powder.
Instant Nonfat Dry Milk Powder	3.6g	4.3	Milk	Contains 0.35 g protein per gm of powder. May be added to food or formula to increase protein and calorie content. 540 mg Na/100 gm powder. 1260 mg Ca/100 mg powder.
Cornstarch	3.5g	8	Corn	Slow release of carbohydrate. Helpful in certain metabolic disorders to treat hypoglycemia.
MCT oil (Mead Johnson)	7.7 ml	14	Lipid fraction of Coconut Oil	Mainly triglycerides of the C_9 and C_{10} saturated fatty acids. Absorbed directly into portal system. Bile salts and lipase not necessary for digestion and absorption. Does not contain essential fatty acids. Non-emulsified, so not recommended for long-term continuous drip feeds.
Corn oil	8.4/ml	14	Corn	Consists primarily of oleic and linoleic unsaturated fatty acids. Non-emulsified, so not recommended for long-term continuous drip feeds.

Table 41. (*continued*)
Infant Carbohydrate-Protein-Fat Modula Additives

Ingredient	Calories	g/Tbsp	Source	Comments
Safflower oil	8.4/ml	14	Safflower	Linoleic and oleic unsaturated fatty acids, non-emulsified, so not recommended for long-term continuous drip feeds.
Microlipid® (Sherwood)	4.5 ml		Safflower oil	50% fat emulsion used as a supplementary source of calories. High in linoleic acid.
Dry Infant Rice Cereal	4.23g	3.5	Rice	May be added to formula to thicken and increase carbohydrate content. Suggest 1 Tbsp/oz maximum. 1 Tbsp = 15 kcal, 0.3 gm protein.
Enfamil Human Milk® Fortifier (Mead Johnson)	14 in 4 packets		Corn syrup solids, Whey protein, Sodium caseinate	For addition to human milk to increase calories, protein Ca, P, Na, vitamins, other minerals, and trace elements. Add 2 pkt/100ml for 24 hr and next day increase to 4 pkt/ 100 ml for full fortification. *See "Formulations Designed for Low Birth Weight Infants."

Table 42.
Average Protein and Calorie Content of Strained Baby Foods*

Product	Amount	Weight (g)	Measure	Calories (tbsp)	Protein (g)	Fat (g)	NA (mg)
Dry infant cereal	1 tbsp	3.6	1	15	0.3	0.1	1
Vegetables	4 oz jar	113	9	50	2.0	0.15	36
Fruits	4 oz jar	113	9	65	0.45 or 0.5	0.09	6.7
Meats	2.5 oz jar	71	5	80	9.0	4	42
Egg Yolk	2 14 oz jars	64	4.5	130	6.0	11	25

*Compiled from data supplied by Gerber Products Company, Fremont, Michigan, 1991.

Table 43.
Drug-Nutrient Interactions

I. Drugs may interfere with nutrient absorption or metabolism by several mechanisms. For example, metronidazole may alter taste sensations. Penicillamine, clofibrate, amphetamines, cytotoxic agents, anticholinergics, and digoxin (toxic levels), may cause anorexia. Cyproheptadine, phenothiazines, benzodiazepines, tricyclic antidepressants, hypoglycemic agents and corticosteroids may cause hyperphagia.

II. The following list offers a few examples where drugs may induce specific nutritional deficiencies or toxicities. The list is not meant to be all-inclusive.

A. Cholestyramine	Malabsorption of vitamins, A, D, K, and folate
Clofibrate	
Colestipol	
B. Colchicine	Vitamin B_{12} deficiency
Rapid potassium repletion	
C. Methotrexate	Folate deficiency
Sulfasalazine	
Trimethoprim	
Triamterene	
Oral contraceptives	
Phenytoin	
Ethanol	also vitamin B, and B_{12} deficiency
D. Isoniazid	Pyridoxine (vitamin B_6) deficiency
Hydralazine	isoniazid also associated with tryptophan and niacin deficiency
Cycloserine	
Ethionamide	
Penicillamine	
L-dopa	

Table 43. (*continued*)
Drug-Nutrient Interactions

Oral contraceptives	
Aspirin	
Barbiturates	
Phenytoin	
E. Antibiotics	Vitamin K deficiency
F. Antacids	Vitamin D deficiency
Laxatives	
Phenytoin	
Barbiturates	
G. Salicylates	Iron deficiency
Antacids	
H_2 blockers	
H. Amphotericin Diuretics	Hypokalemia, Hypomagnesemia
Diuretics	also hyponatremia
Cisplatin	
Cyclosporin	also hypertriglyceridemia
I. Steroids	Hyperglycemia
L-asparaginase	
J. Pentamidine	Hypoglycemia
K. Sucralfate	Hypophosphatemia
Steroids	
antacids	
L. Thiazide diuretics	Hypercalcemia
M. Nanthiazide diuretics	Hypocalcemia
	Probenecid

Table 44.
Laboratory Values During Pregnancy

Laboratory Test	Normal Values		Findings in Deficiency During Pregnancy
	Non-pregnant	Pregnant	
Urinary acetone	Neg	Faint pos in am	Positive
Serum total protein (g/100 ml)	6.5–8.5	6–8	>6
Serum alb (g/100 ml)	3.5–5	2.5–4.5	<3.5
BUN (mg/100 ml)	10–25	5–15	<5
Fasting glucose (mg/100 ml)	70–110	65–100	<65
2hr Postprandial glucose (mg/100 ml)	<100	<120 (plasma)	>120
Serum Ca (mEq/l)	4.6–5.5	4.2–5.2	<4.2 or normal
Serum P (mg/100 ml)	2.5–4.8	2.3–4.6	No change
Alk Phos (IU/l)	35–180	35–180	No change
Chol (mg/100 ml)	120–290	177–355	N/A
TG (mg/100 ml)	33–166	130–400	N/A
Serum folate (ng/ml)	5–21	4–14	<4
Vit B_{12} (pg/ml)	430–1025	Decreased	Decreased
Serum Fe (μg/ml)	>50	>60	<60
TIBC μg/100/ml)	250–400	300–600	<450
% TIBC sat.	30	≥20	<16
Serum Zn (μg/100 ml)	65–115	55–80	±50
Urinary Zn (μg/day)	200–450	200–450	±150

Adapted from Aubrey RH, Roberts A and Ceunca VG: The assessment of maternal nutrition. Clin Perinatal 1975;2:207–19.

Table 45.
Sodium Content of Selected Medications*

Drug	mg	mEq
Aminosalicylate Sodium, 1 g	108.7	4.7
Ampicillin Sodium, 1 g	66.7	2.9
Ampicillin Sodium, 1 g and Sulbactam, 0.5 g	115.0	5.0
Azlocillin Sodium, 1 g	50.0	2.17
Carbenicillin Disodium, 1 g	108.1–121.9	4.7–5.3†
Cefazolin Sodium, 1 g	46.0–48.3	2.0–2.1
Cefaperazone Sodium, 1 g	34.0	1.5
Cefotaxime Sodium, 1 g	50.5	2.2
Cefotetan Disodium, 1 g	80.0	3.5
Cefoxitin Sodium, 1 g	53.8	2.3
Ceftazidime, 1 g	53.8	2.3
Ceftizoxime Sodium, 1 g	60.0	2.6
Ceftriaxone Sodium, 1 g	82.8	3.6
Cefuroxime Sodium, 1 g	54.2	2.4
Chloramphenicol Sodium Succinate, 1 g	51.8	2.3
Methicillin Sodium, 1 g	66.7	2.9
Mezlocillin Sodium, 1 g	42.6	1.85
Moxalactam Sodium, 1 g	88.0	3.8
Nafcillin Sodium, 1 g	66.7	2.9
Oxacillin Sodium, 1 g	64.4	2.8
Penicillin G Potassium, 1 million units	7.6	0.3
Penicillin G Sodium, 1 million units	46.0	2.0
Phenytoin Sodium, 1 g	88.0	3.8
Piperacillin Sodium, 1 g	42.6	1.85
Sodium Bicarbonate, 50 ml of 7.5%, 8.4%	1026, 1150	44.6, 50.06
Sodium Iodide, 1 g	156.0	.8
Sodium Polystyrene Sulfonate, 1 g, oral	94.3‡	4.1‡
Thiopental Sodium, 1 g	86.8	3.8
Ticarcillin Disodium, 1 g	119.6†	5.2†
Ticarcillin Disodium and Clavulanate Potassium, 1 g	109	4.75

*Product formulation and sodium content are subject to change by manufacturer.
†Sodium content per gram of free acid; actual vial content can be as high as 6.5 mEq/g.
‡Total sodium content; only approximately 33% is liberated in clinical use.
Knoben JE, Anderson PO, eds. Handbook of Clinical Drug Data, 6th Ed. Drug Intelligence Publ, Hamilton, IL, 1988 and Parenteral and Enteral Nutrition Handbook (UCLA Medical Center).

APPENDIX 2

Growth Charts

Figure 1.
Girls: Birth to 36 months physical growth NCHS percentiles

(Adapted from Hamill PV, Drizd TA, Johnson CL, et al. Physical growth: National Center for Health Statistics percentiles. Am J Clin Nutr 1979:32:607–629. Am J Clin Nutr American Society for Clinical Nutrition. Data from the Fels Longitudinal Study, Wright State University School of Medicine, Yellow Springs, Ohio).

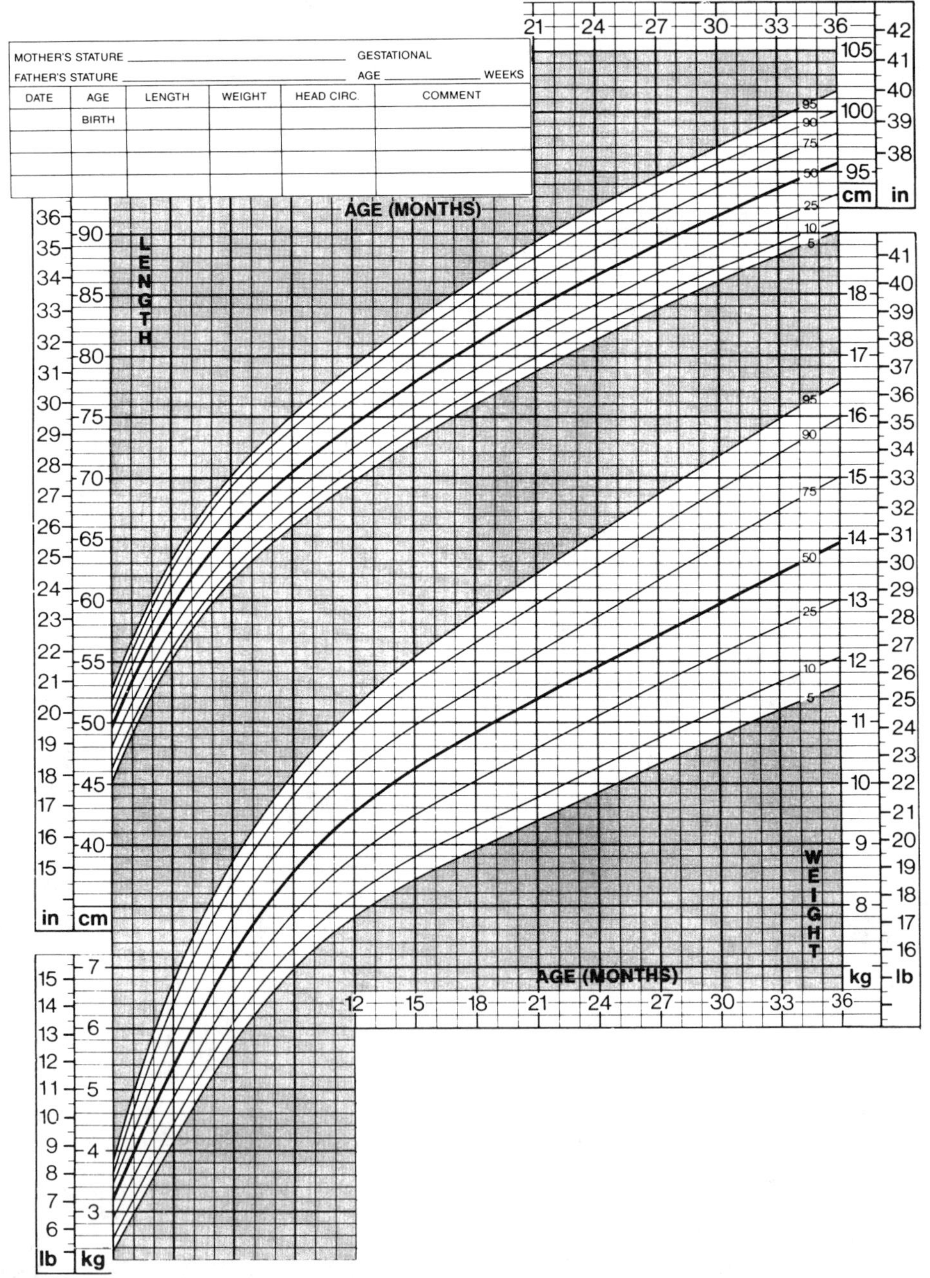

Figure 2.

Girls: 2 to 18 years physical growth NCHS percentiles.

(Adapted from Hamill PV, Drizd TA, Johnson CL, et al. Physical growth: National Center for Health Statistics percentiles. Am J Clin Nutr 1979:32:607–629. Am J Clin Nutr American Society for Clinical Nutrition. Data from the National Center for Health Statistics (NCHS), Hyattsville, Maryland).

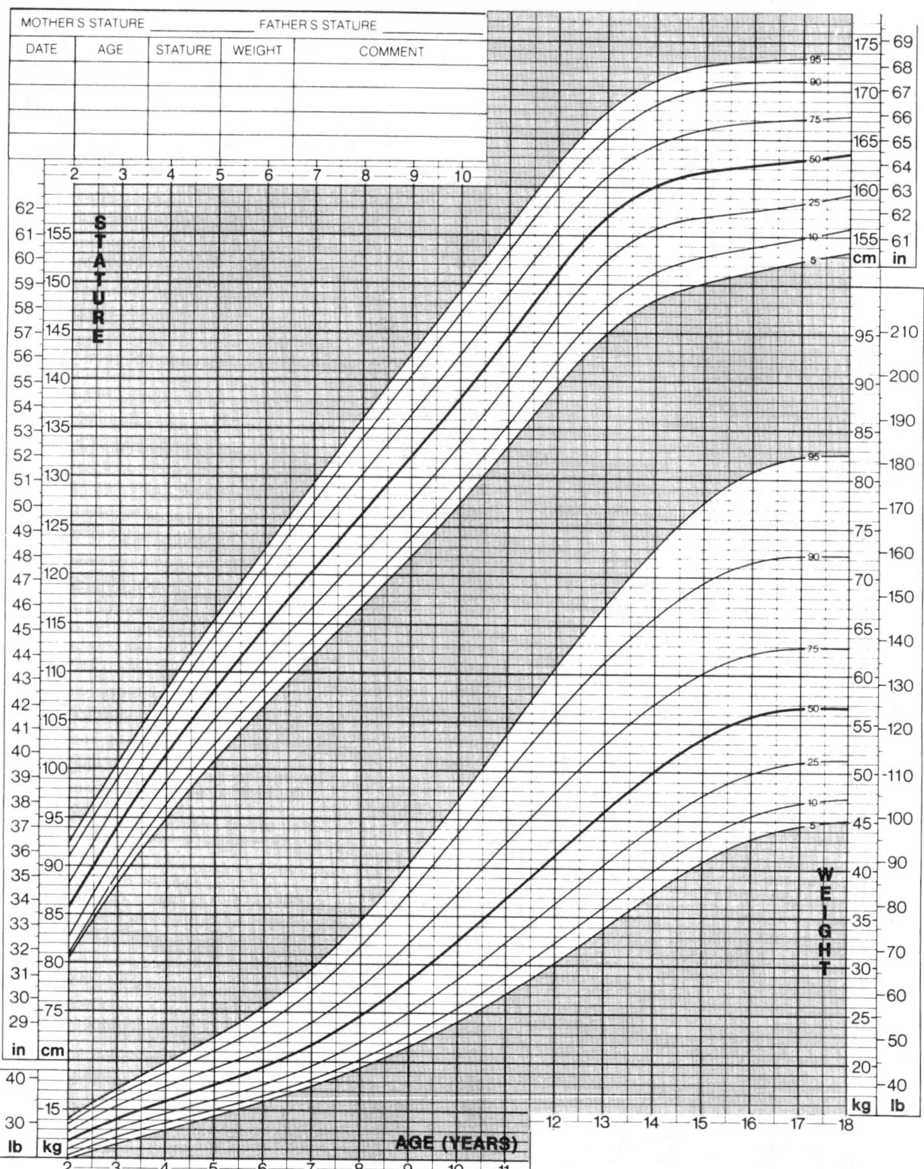

Figure 3.

Boys: Birth to 36 months physical growth NCHS percentiles.

(Adapted from Hamill PV, Drizd TA, Johnson CL, et al. Physical growth: National Center for Health Statistics percentiles. Am J Clin Nutr 1979:32:607–629. Am J Clin Nutr American Society for Clinical Nutrition. Data from the Fels Longitudinal Study, Wright State University School of Medicine, Yellow Springs, Ohio).

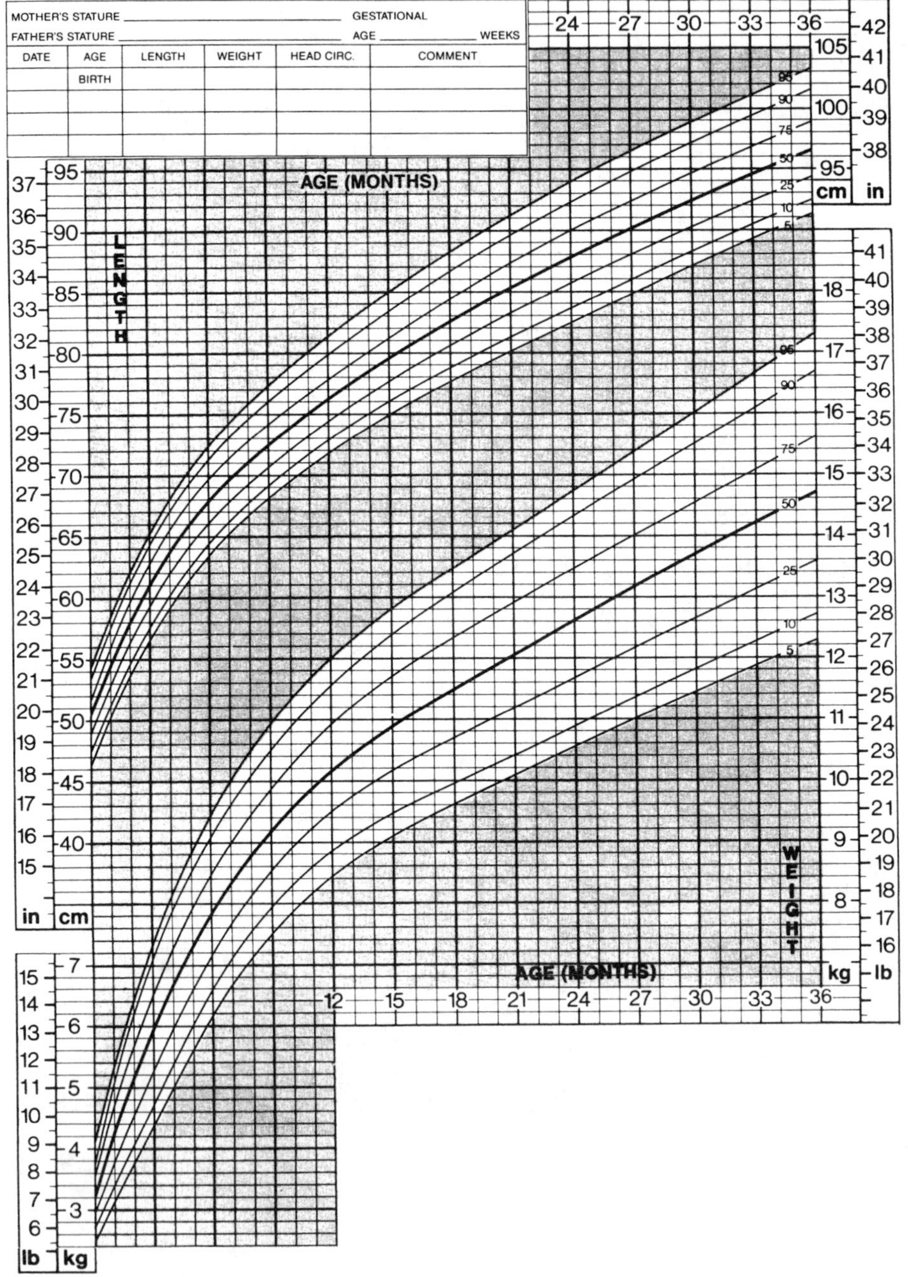

Figure 4.
Boys: 2 to 18 years physical growth, NCHS percentiles.

(Adapted from Hamill PV, Drizd TA, Johnson CL, et al. Physical growth: National Center for Health Statistics percentiles. Am J Clin Nutr 1979:32:607–629. Am J Clin Nutr American Society for Clinical Nutrition. Data from the National Center for Health Statistics (NCHS), Hyattsville, Maryland).

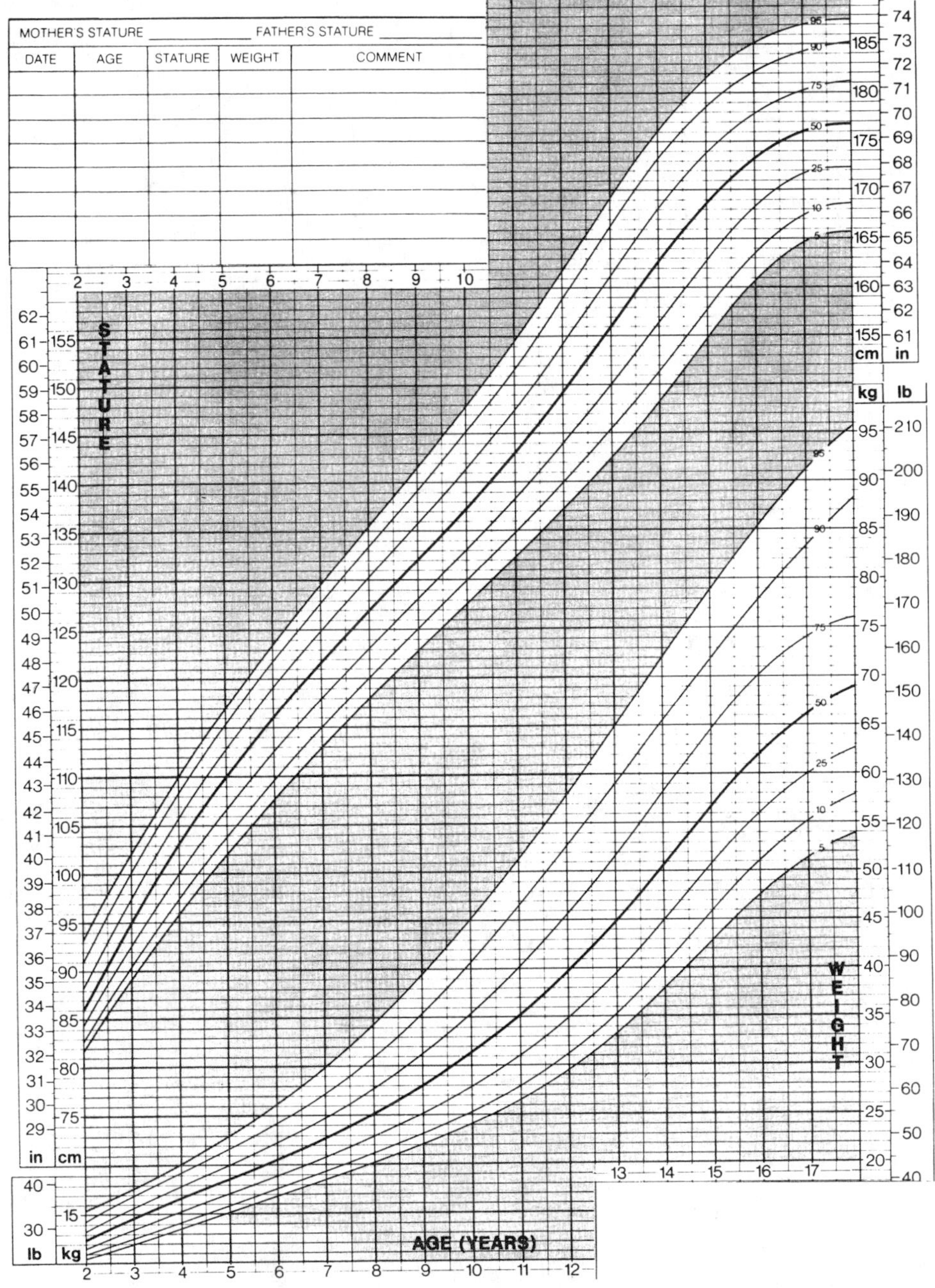

Figure 5.
Height velocity, girls.

(Reprinted with permission from Tanner JM, Davis PSW. Clinical longitudinal standards for height and height velocity for North American children. J Peds 1985; 107:317–329.).

Patient's Name | Birth Date

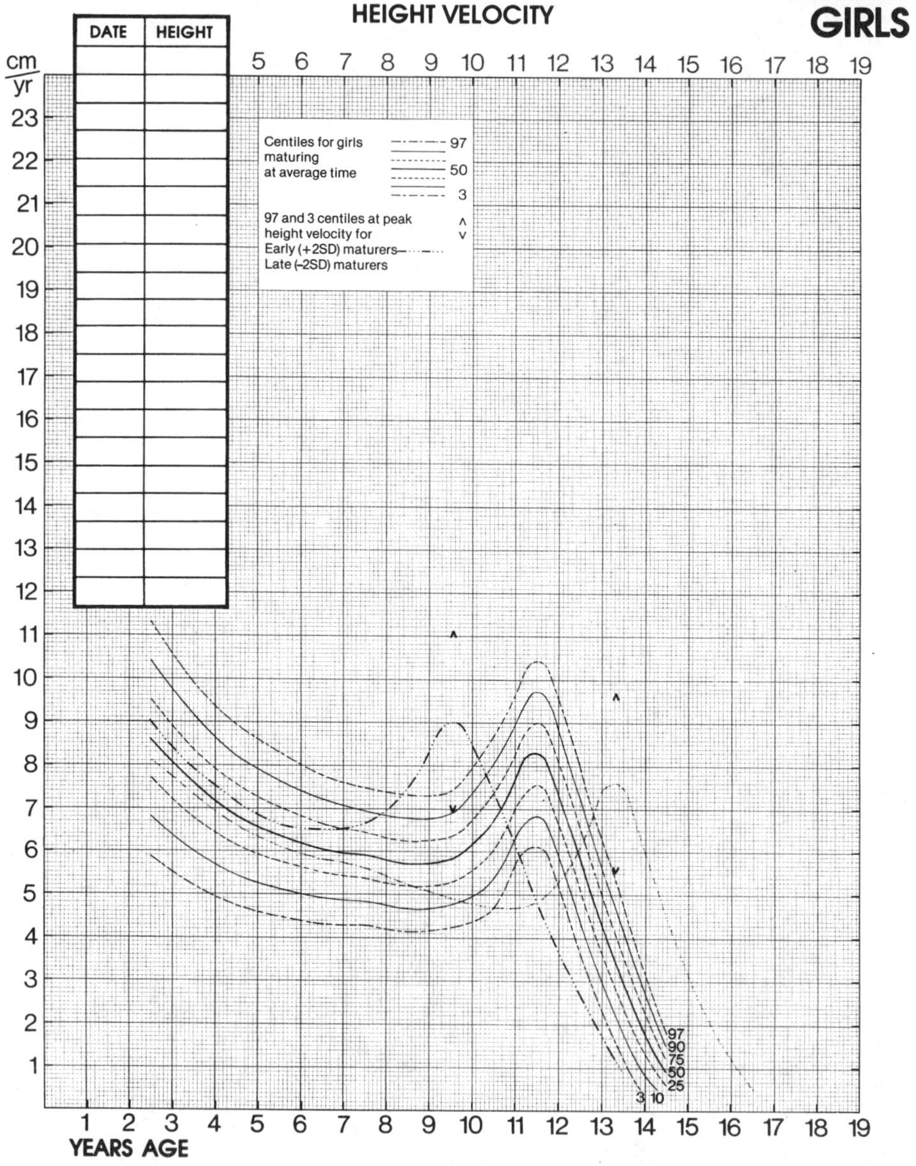

Figure 6.
Height velocity, boys.

(Reprinted with permission from Tanner JM, Davis PSW. J Peds 1985;107).

Patient's Name | Birth Date

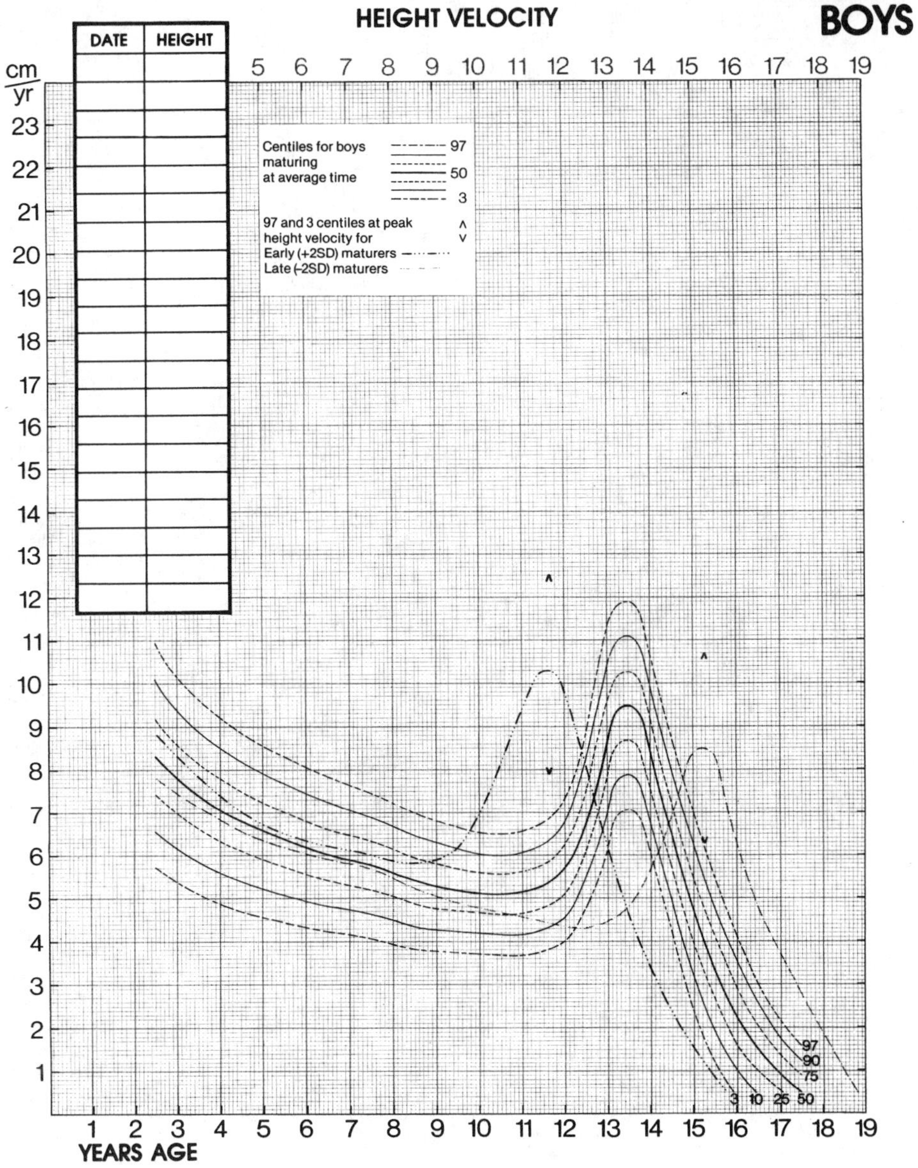

Figure 7.
Weight velocity, girls.

(Reprinted with permission from Tanner JM, Whitehouse RH. Pediatric Gastrointestinal Disease—Pathophysiology, Diagnosis, Management. Wyllie/Hyams, 1993).

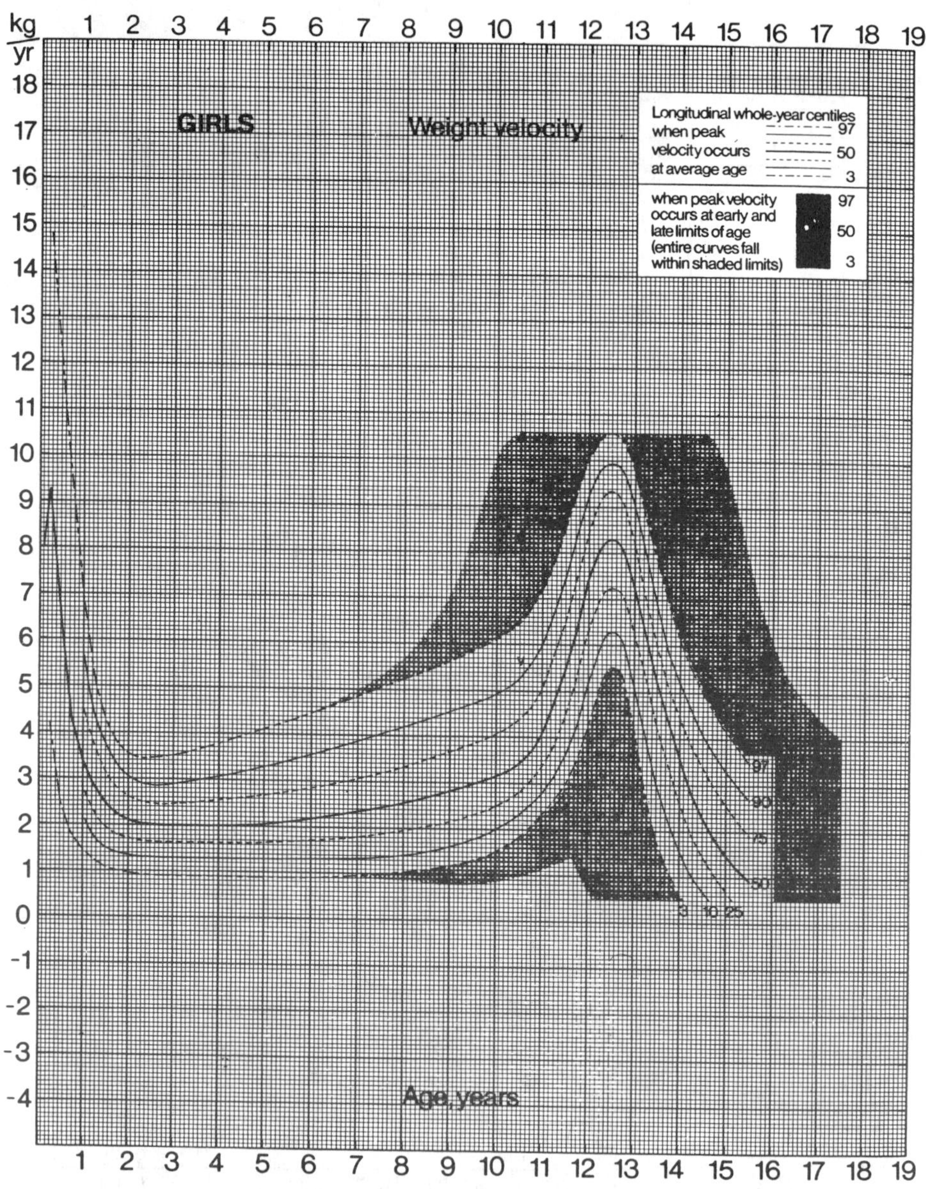

Figure 8.
Weight velocity, boys.

(Reprinted with permission from Tanner JM, Whitehouse RH. Pediatric Gastrointestinal Disease—Pathophysiology, Diagnosis, Management. Wyllie/Hyams, 1993).

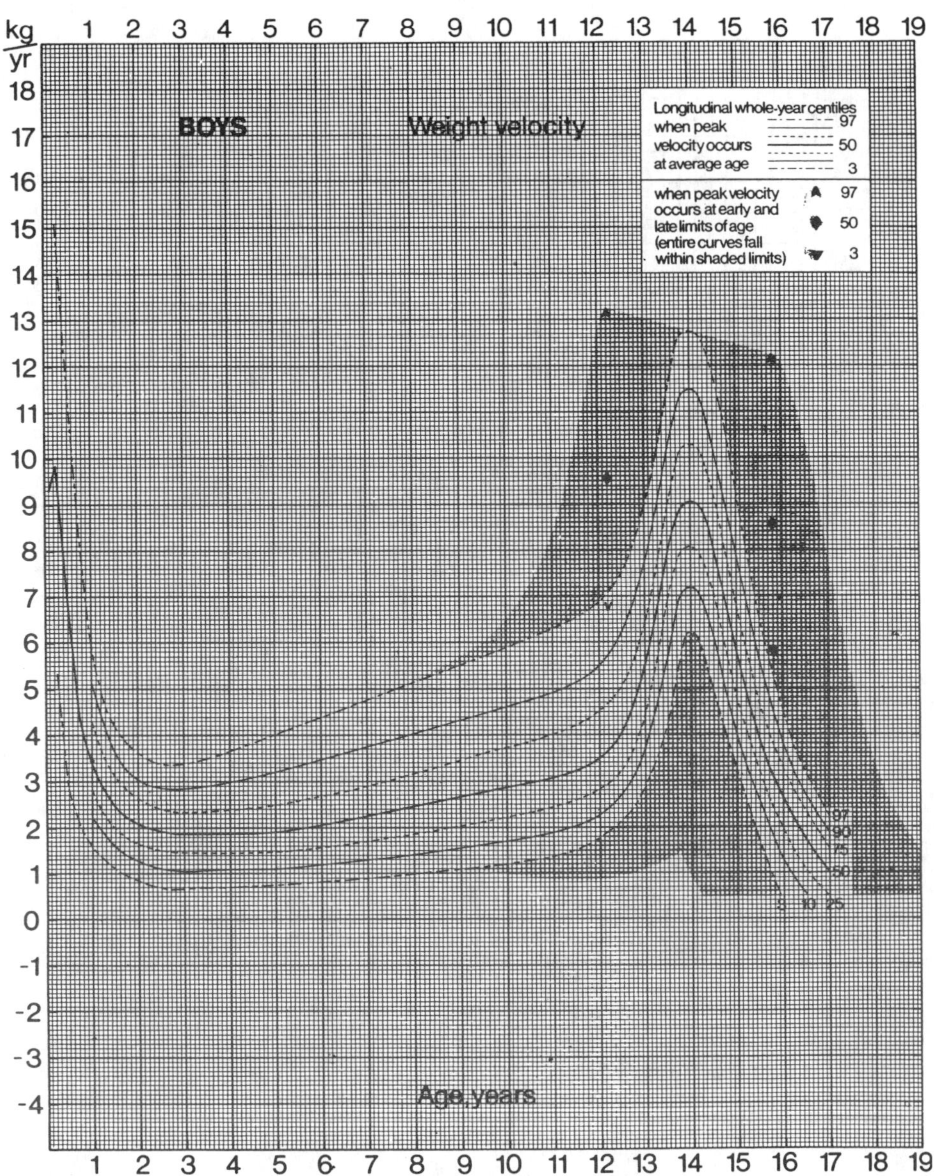

Figure 9.

Perinatal growth chart at gestational age. Combined intrauterine-neonatal growth chart for length, weight, and OFC.

(Adapted from Lubcheno, et al. Pediatrics 1966;37:403, and from Children's Med Center, Boston—Anthropometric Chart).

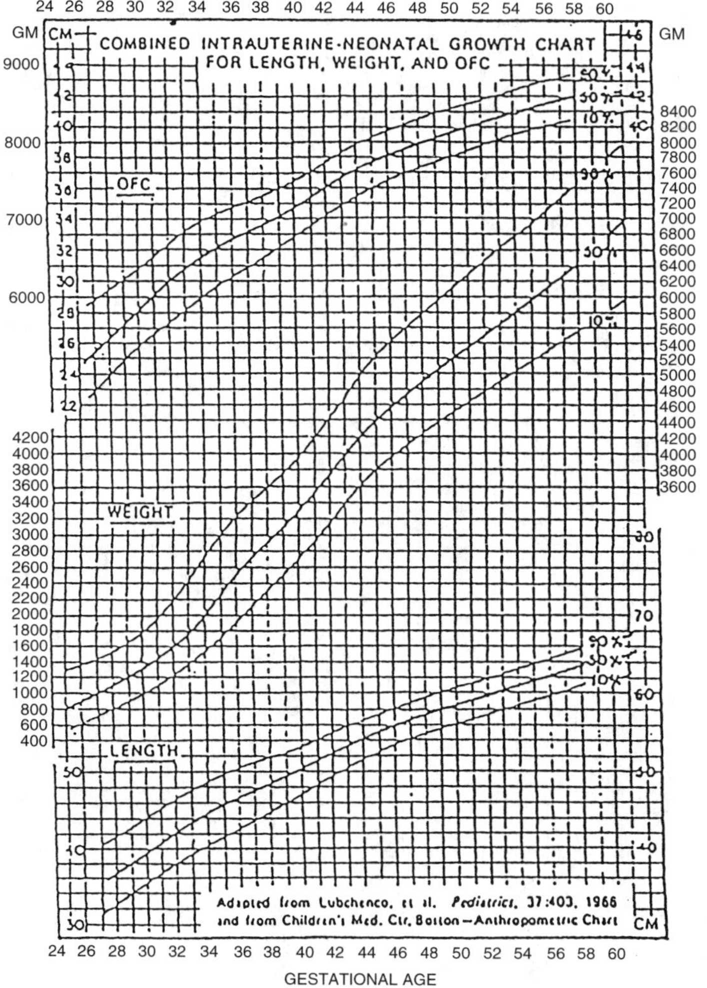

Figure 10.
Intrauterine length chart. Both sexes. Fetal body length percentiles from 28 to 43 weeks of gestation.

(Reprinted with permission from Naeye RL, Dixon JB. Distortions in fetal growth standards. Pediatr Res 1978;12:987–1003.)

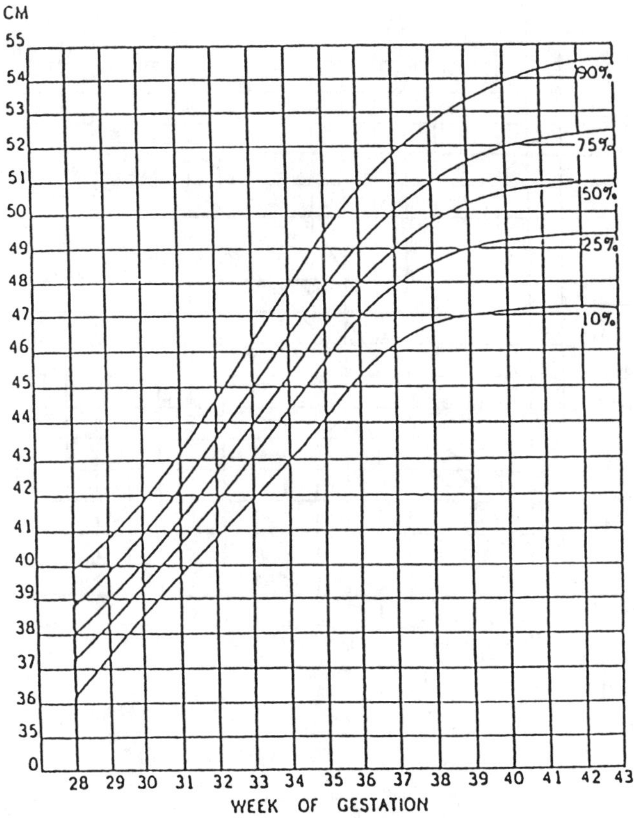

Figure 11.
Intrauterine weight chart. Both sexes. Fetal weight percentiles from 28 to 43 weeks of gestation.

(Reprinted with permission from Naeye RL, Dixon JB. Distortions in fetal growth standards. Pediatr Res 1978;12:987–1003.)

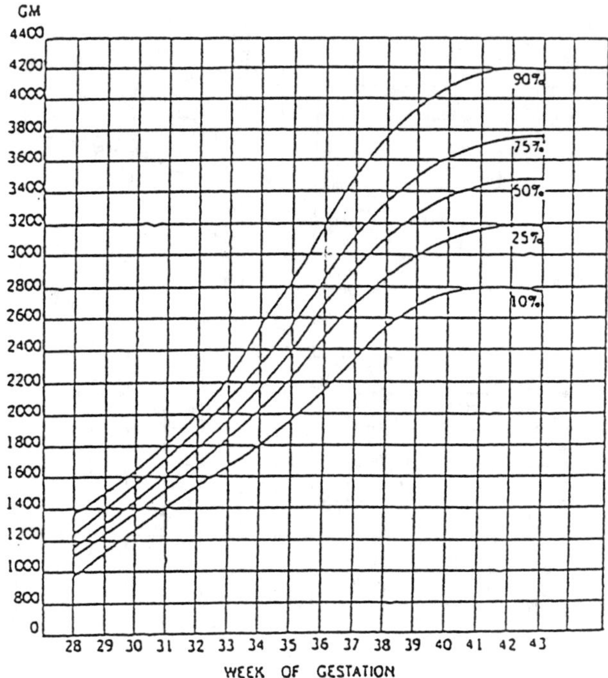

Figure 12.

Down syndrome, height and weight for girls, 1 to 36 months.

(Reprinted with permission from Cronk C, Crocker AC, Siegfried M, et al. Growth charts for children with Down syndrome: 1 month to 18 years of age. Pediatrics 1988;81:102–110).

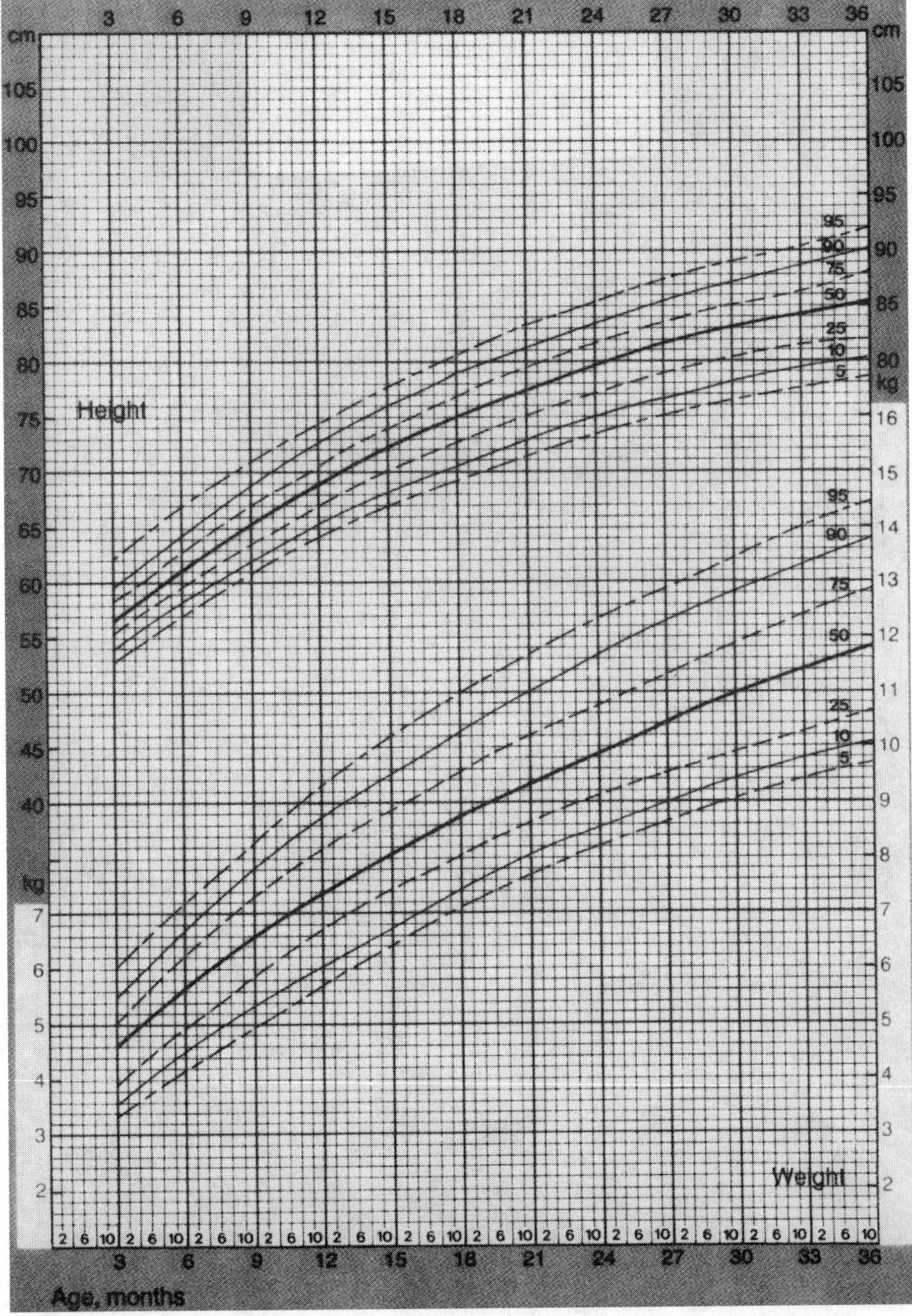

Figure 13.
Down syndrome, height and weight for boys, 1 to 36 months.

(Reprinted with permission from Cronk C, Crocker AC, Siegfried M, et al. Growth charts for children with Down syndrome: 1 month to 18 years of age. Pediatrics 1988;81:102–110).

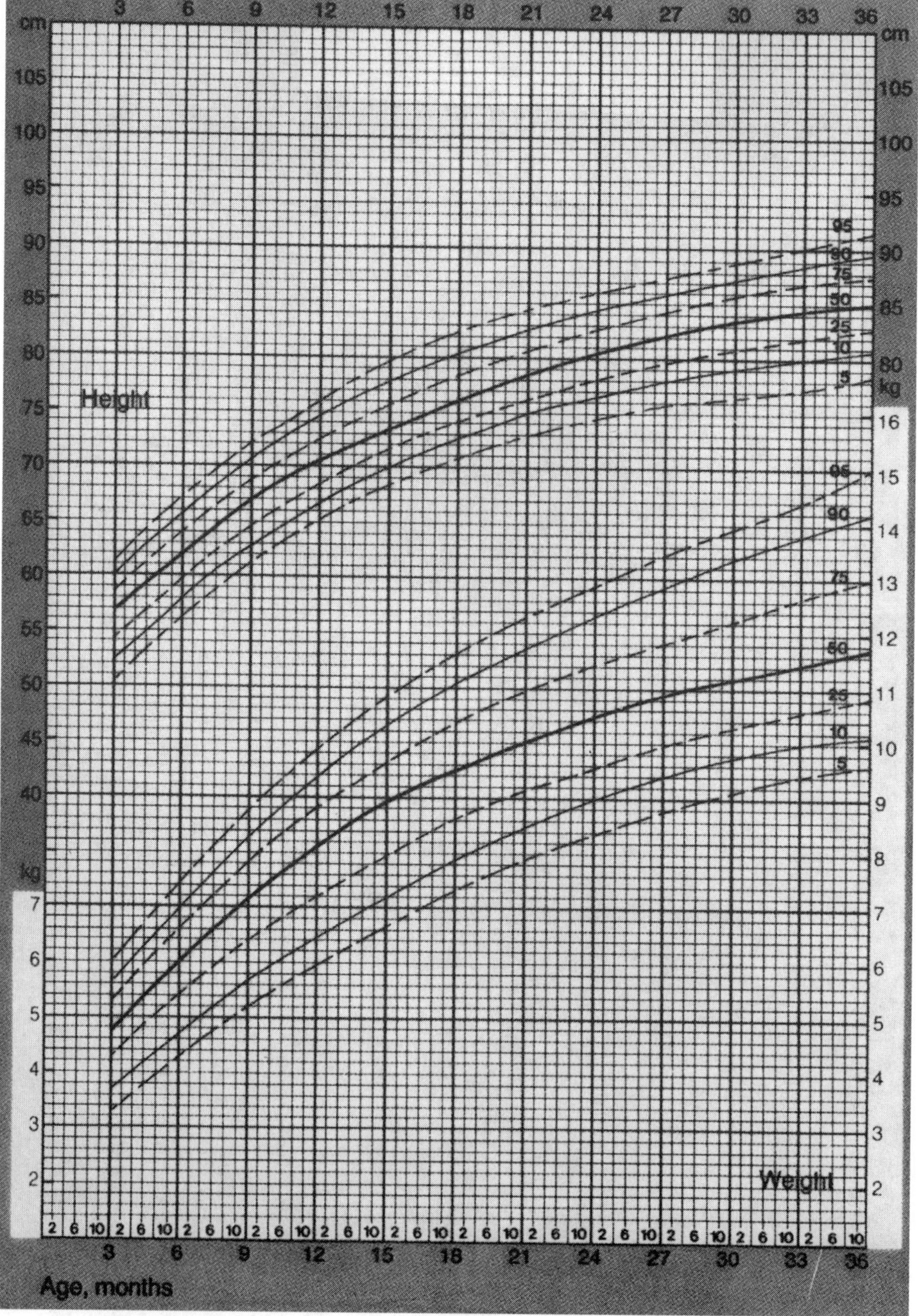

Figure 14.
Down syndrome, height and weight for girls, 2 to 18 years.

(Reprinted with permission from Cronk C, Crocker AC, Siegfried M, et al. Growth charts for children with Down syndrome: 1 month to 18 years of age. Pediatrics 1988;81:102–110).

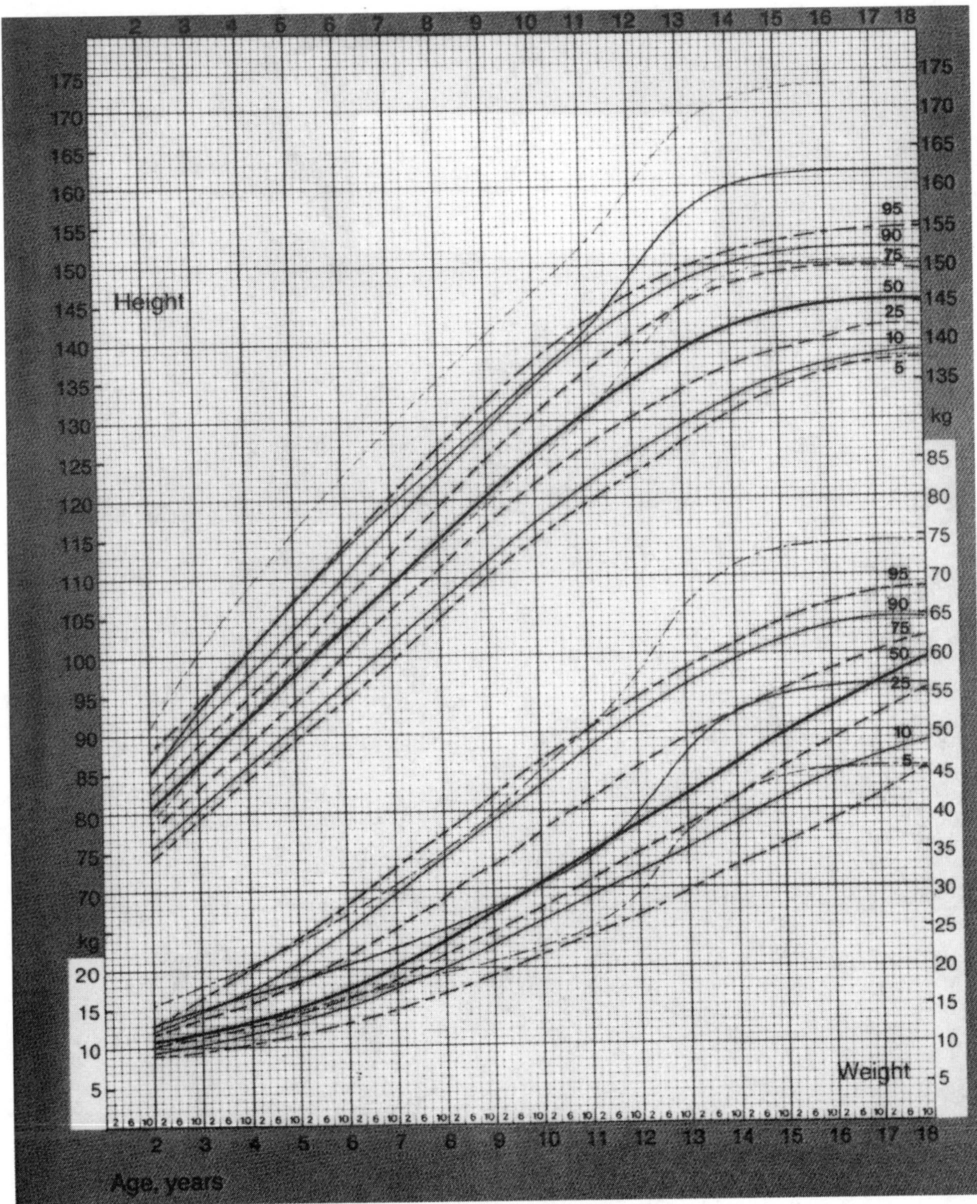

Figure 15.

Down syndrome, height and weight for boys, 2 to 18 years.

(Reprinted with permission from Cronk C, Crocker AC, Siegfried M, et al. Growth charts for children with Down syndrome: 1 month to 18 years of age. Pediatrics 1988;81:102–110).

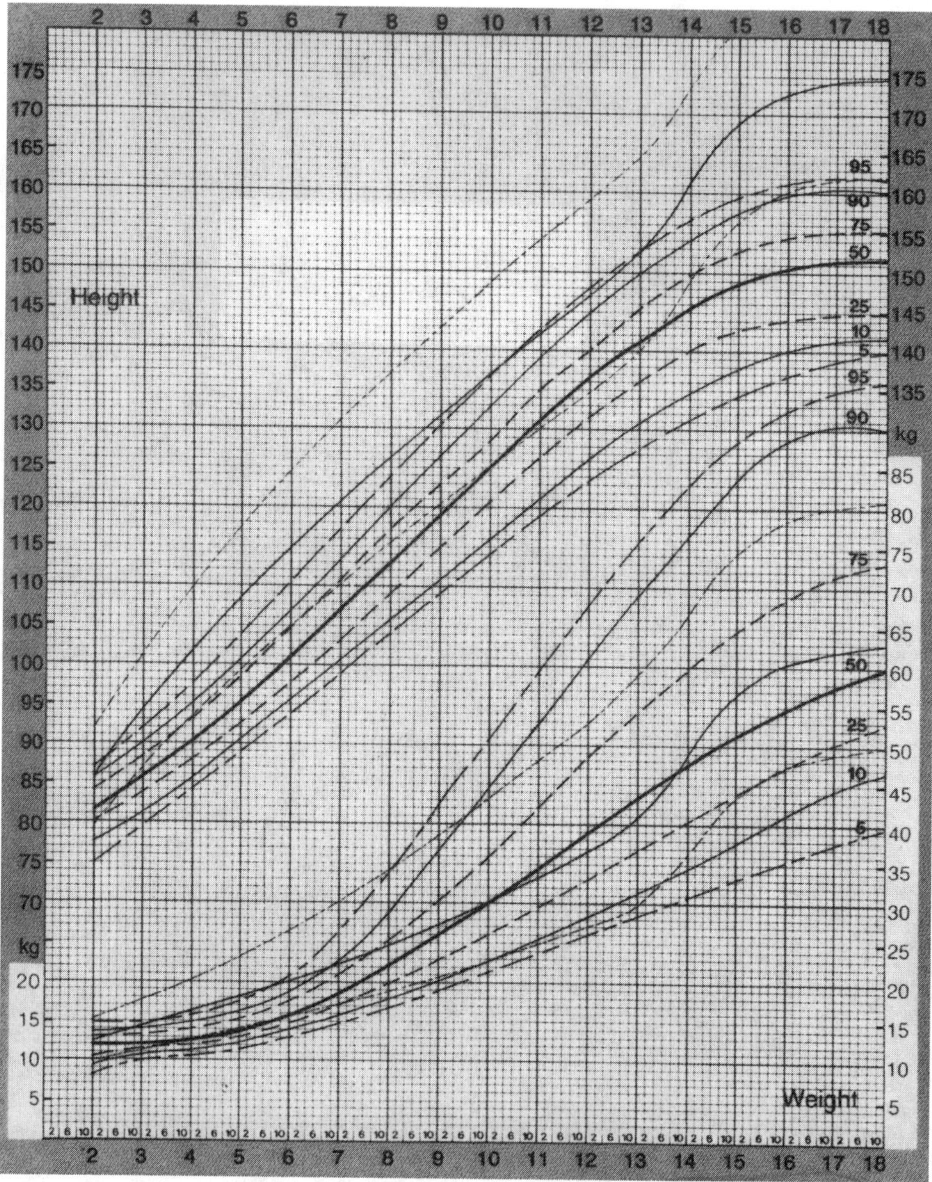

Figure 16.
Girls: birth to 36 months physical growth NCHS percentiles.

(Adapted from Hamill PV, Drizd TA, Johnson CL, et al. Physical growth: National Center for Health Statistics percentiles. Am J Clin Nutr 1979;32:607–629. Data from the Fels Longitudinal Study, Wright State University School of Medicine, Yellow Springs, Ohio).

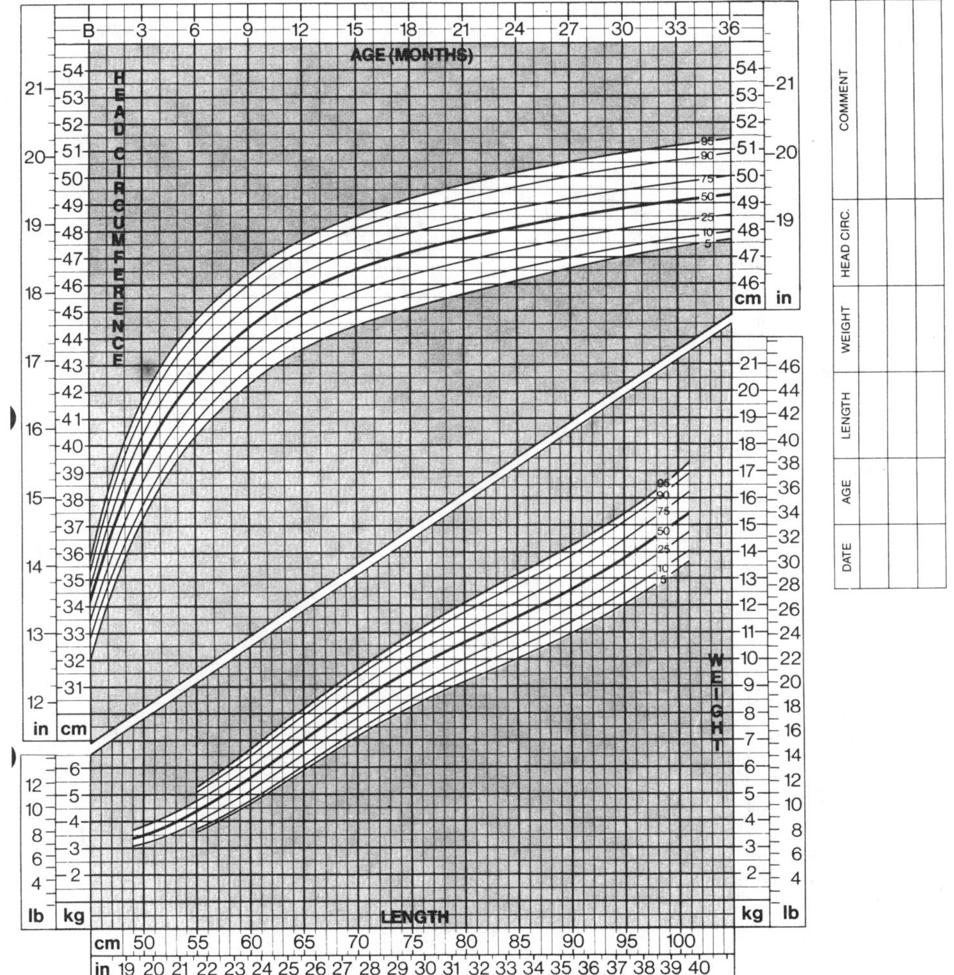

Figure 17.
Girls: prepubescent physical growth NCHS percentiles.

(Adapted from Hamill PV, Drizd TA, Johnson CL, et al. Physical growth: National Center for Health Statistics percentiles. Am J Clin Nutr 1979;32:607–629. Data from the National Center for Health Statistics (NCHS), Hyattsville, Maryland).

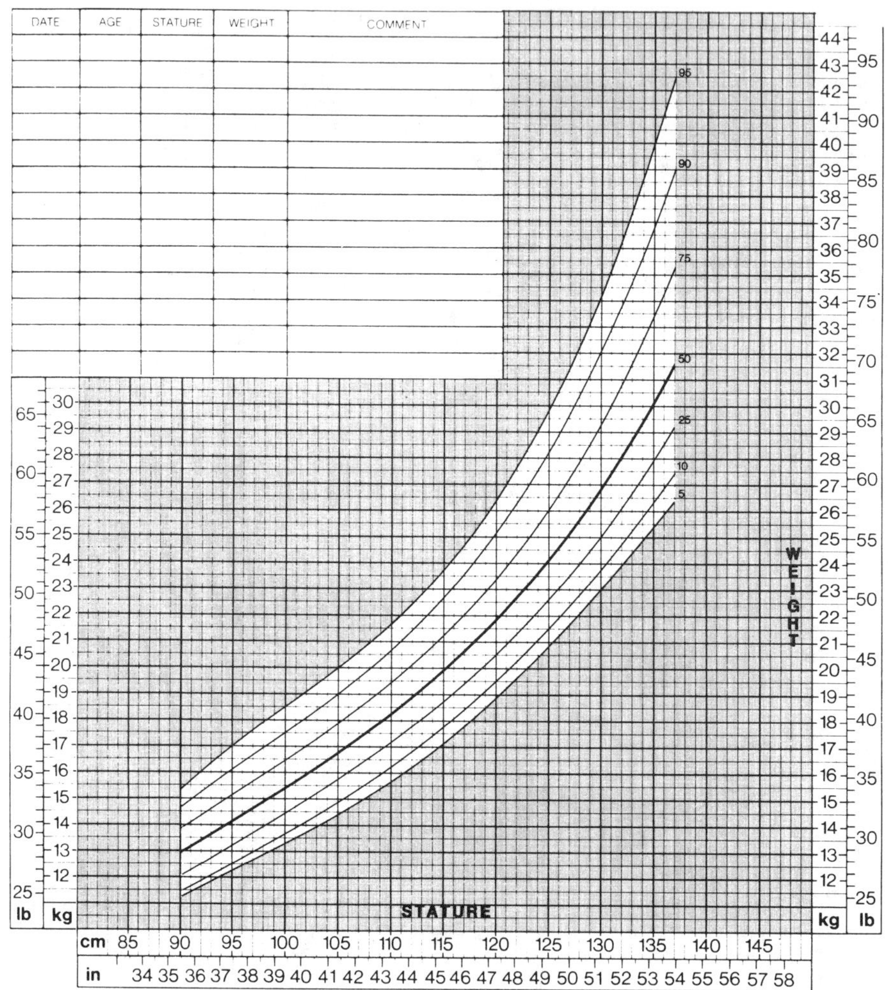

Figure 18.

Boys: birth to 36 months physical growth NCHS percentiles.

(Adapted from Hamill PV, Drizd TA, Johnson CL, et al. Physical growth: National Center for Health Statistics percentiles. Am J Clin Nutr 1979;32:607–629. Data from the Fels Longitudinal Study, Wright State University School of Medicine, Yellow Springs, Ohio).

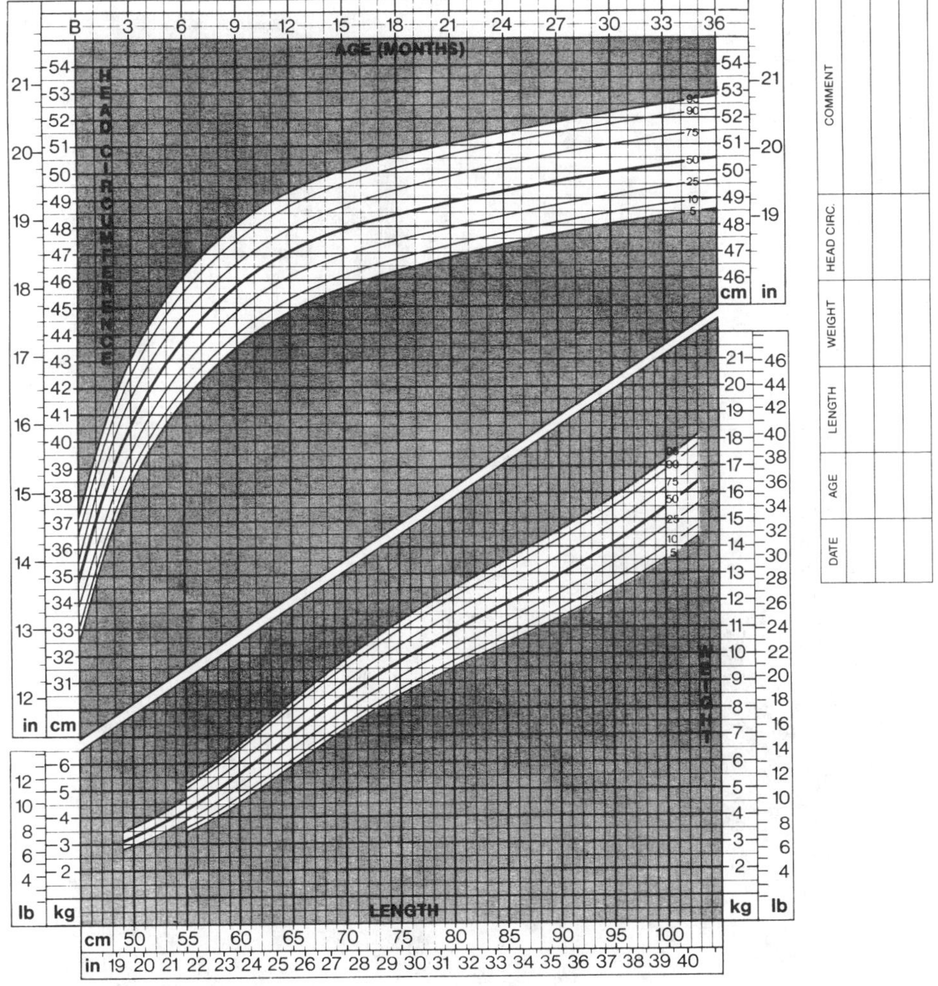

Figure 19.

Boys: prepubescent physical growth NCHS percentiles.

(Adapted from Hamill PV, Drizd TA, Johnson CL, et al. Physical growth: National Center for Health Statistics percentiles. Am J Clin Nutr 1979;32:607–629. Data from the National Center for Health Statistics (NCHS), Hyattsville, Maryland).

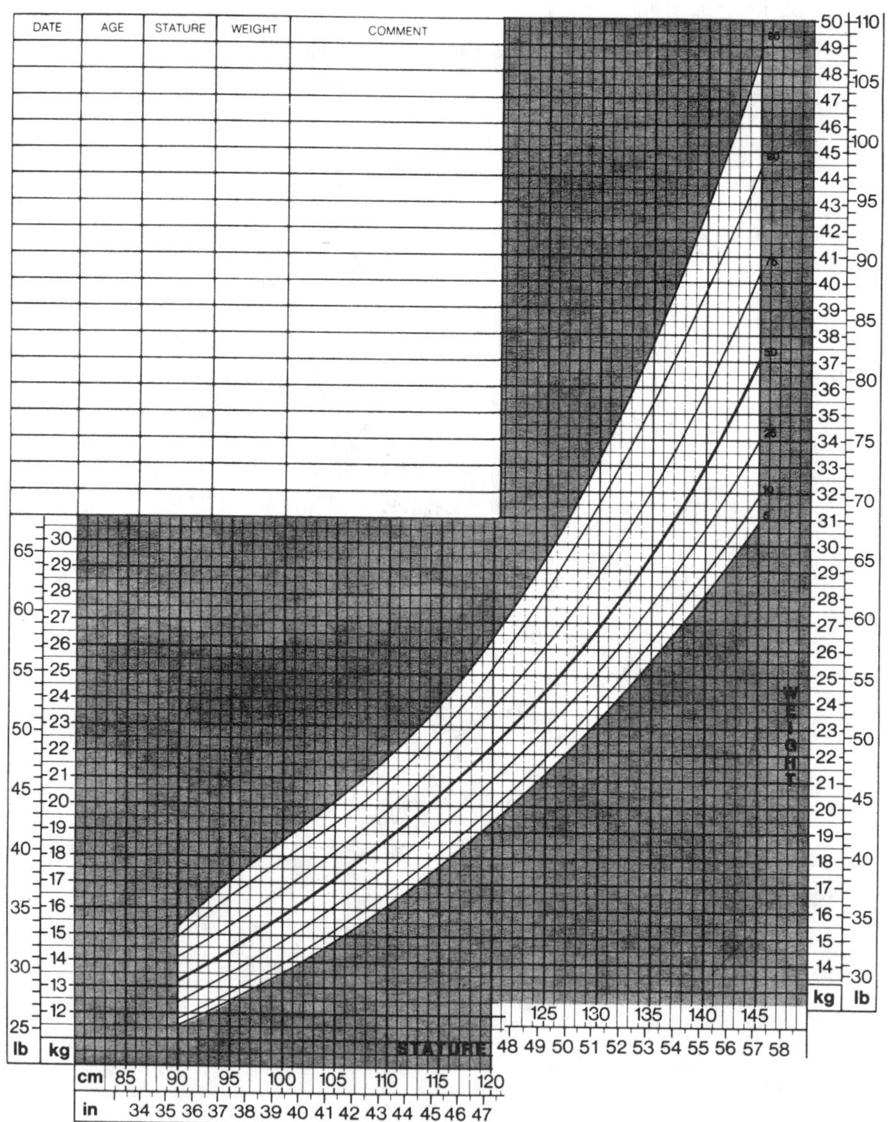

Figure 20.

Head circumference in centimeters. Classification of newborns based on maturity and intrauterine growth.

(Adapted from Lubchenco LO, Hansman C, Boyd E. Pediatrics 1966;37:403 and Battaglia FC, Lubchenco LO. J Pediatr 1967;71:159).

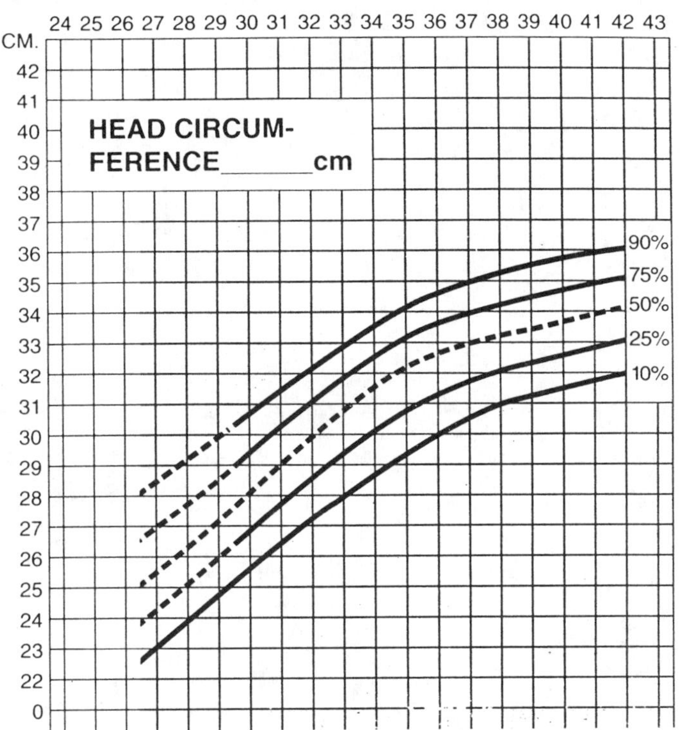

Index

Page numbers in *italics* refer to illustrations; page numbers followed by t refer to tables.